Foreword

In Yoga Journey, Becky Pell offers you a clear and practical guide to the timeless wisdom of yoga and how it can help you. With the warm and welcoming tone characteristic of her teaching, Becky's love for yoga and its gifts shines through in this valuable addition to your practice.

Becky and I first met on the mat at my long-standing studio 'The Yoga Hutch' in London. She popped her mat quietly in the corner and began an astoundingly mindful practice. After a few visits we gradually began to get to know one another and our friendship has been one of those wonderful 'slow-grow' friendships that time and experience have told me are the ones that last.

It's fascinating to observe people as they arrive in my studio and become absorbed in the special energy and community we have created. The Yoga Hutch is a small space with a huge heart, and we have a dedicated community of practitioners that have stayed with us for years. My teaching has inspired many people to find clarity and purpose in their lives and our sanctuary has brought a community together even in the trickiest of times. I am practical by nature - give me something broken, whether it's a chair or a person and I will fix it! I practised as an architect before I switched to yoga; and whilst these skills are seemingly miles apart, when we are true to ourselves, recognise our skills and embrace our innate talents we flourish and can be the best version of ourselves.

A little enigmatic when she first joined the Yoga Hutch community, Becky would come along and practice quietly in her corner very regularly for weeks at a time and then disappear off for months as she toured the world as a sound engineer.

There was something about her that fascinated me from the start -she was reserved and very composed, yet the crazy leggings and beautiful tattoos expressed what I could see in her eyes and in her practice… that she was so much more!

She kept coming back, and as our post-class conversations grew, I realised that not only did she spend much of her life on the road as a sound engineer, but also had undergone yoga teacher training. We began to practice together and so grew a real relationship of trust and connection.

Becky joined my teacher mentoring program and before I knew it the mentoring was two-way traffic. She taught many of my classes and helped me understand myself a little more along the way. Her knowledge and depth of understanding of the expansive nature of yoga as an all-encompassing way of living is truly authentic and natural for her. Becky is a teacher of worldliness and intelligence, as well as an accredited yoga therapist, sound engineer, and writer.

Nothing deters Becky from hard work and embracing change. When she moved to Australia, we quickly realised that we could continue to work and collaborate by running yoga retreats together. Our 'Find Your Balance' retreats began and have flourished into a wonderful international and 'at home' retreat business. These have been an amazing connection for us both, and our students love Becky's blissfully restorative classes and profound yoga wisdom.

Our friendship has grown into one that transcends time, space and distance and Becky's wisdom, love and enthusiasm for life and yoga is a beaming light that shines through in her writing.

Yoga Journey – a Contemporary Guide to a Timeless Tradition is a breath of fresh air. In these pages you will find a clear and concise description of an enormous subject that can otherwise take years to grasp. The words are economical and precise where they need to be, and explain many complex concepts within yoga philosophy without avoiding the difficult 'stuff'. Becky's candid nature and humour are apparent in her writing, and her clear uncomplicated perspective enables a deeper understanding with an extraordinary relevance to the lives we live today.

With the mind of an engineer, the perspective of a yoga therapist, and the heart of a devoted yogi and meditator, Becky has created a travel guide for your own yoga journey. This is a book for everyone who suspects that there's a path to more inspired living and would like a little light shining on the road ahead.

This easy-to-read book provides a valuable insight into yoga as a whole, both on and off the mat. It will show you how the ancient wisdom of yoga can inform, enrich and illuminate every aspect of your day-to day-life, helping you to navigate challenges with greater grace, ease and steadiness. You will learn not only effective ways to develop different aspects of your yoga practice, but also how and why they work.

This book will inform and inspire you. A gem solidly grounded in extensive study and supported by years of dedicated practice and teaching, *Yoga Journey* makes it easy to understand how we can all use the vast wealth of yoga's wisdom to make our own lives a better place to be.

Yoga Journey is an accessible, practical gathering of profound wisdom, thought provoking and applicable to modern living – it is compelling and readable, enormously informative and absolutely essential reading.

Sarah Vaughan, Senior Astanga Yoga Teacher, yoga teacher mentor, life lover, and blessed to be Becky's friend.

3rd September 2020.

Introduction

If you enjoy yoga and are eager to learn more about the practice beyond the postures, this book is for you.

I was inspired to write it after a conversation with a friend who had recently discovered yoga and was considering doing her teacher training to deepen her knowledge and experience. She asked me whether I could recommend any books that might help her to better understand yoga beyond the mat. My first response was 'yes, of course!' Thinking about it later that day, I realised that although there are lots of great books out there about different aspects of yoga, I didn't know of any that would quite fit the bill. I was looking for something that would bridge the gap between studio classes and a teacher training curriculum. Something that explored both the foundational yoga practices and philosophies as well as more advanced concepts, making them accessible and relevant to everyday modern life; something for anyone who wants a better understanding of yoga as a whole; something to get under the skin of what happens on the mat.

I couldn't find what I was looking for, so I decided to write it myself.

The language of yoga is the ancient tongue of Sanskrit. Throughout this book you will see Sanskrit terms in *italics*, alongside their English translation. Sanskrit differentiates between sounds denoted by the letter 's' with the addition of a dot below or dash above the letter, which make a 'sh' sound. The letter 'c' also makes different sounds. To allow for easier reading, I have used the Anglicised phonetic spellings (eg Ashtanga vs Astanga; chakra vs cakra). I have also used the Anglicised addition of an 's' to denote plurals.

Chapter 1 – What *is* Yoga?

Yoga is a comprehensive methodology for living well and looking after all aspects of ourselves. Extending far beyond the postures (although these can be wonderful techniques to help us cultivate better health, more balanced energy and increased self-awareness), yoga gives us a treasure-trove of tools to make our own lives a better place to be – it's about how we live our lives, not just the time we spend on our mats. The ultimate purpose of yoga is to alleviate our suffering, and help us to experience life as it really is without the clouding of all our mental baggage and so reach a state of Self-realisation – the direct experience of our true nature. But what does that actually mean?

How would you respond to the question 'who are you'? You might respond with your name, age, occupation, where you live, whether you're in a relationship, whether you're a parent, what you like to do in your spare time, and so on. Whilst this is a functional way of explaining how we live our lives, is it who we actually are?

These labels, whilst useful in everyday conversation, limit us if we take them literally. You might teach, but you're not only a teacher. You are a teacher when you are teaching, but at other times, when you are not teaching, you are not a teacher. You might have children, but you're not only a parent. You're a lot more than labels could ever describe.

Is your body 'you'? Well, have you been the same person since you were born? Ostensibly you might think 'yes' – after all, you've had the same name and there's been a continuum of development under this identity. But your body today is not the same as it was when you were 6 months old, or 6 years. It isn't the same at 30 as it is at 60. The atoms which make up your body will be different when you die, from when you were born – in fact we undergo a total bodily recycling over every period of seven to ten years. So your body isn't you.

Your mind then – are you your mind? Your mind chats away constantly. It plans, analyses, has thoughts and opinions and makes decisions, expresses itself and generally directs your life. So you must be your mind, right?

Well….. no. Your mind is the central computer which does all of the actions described above and many more. But if you learn to get really quiet, you might begin to notice that you can observe your thoughts as a witness. You can actually sit back and watch the mental events as they arise.

So who is it that is doing the watching?

Aha. *That's* you.

Your true identity is the witness consciousness which is able to observe the mental goings-on as an onlooker. Your self – small 's' – is the collection of labels which you use to describe yourself; your human avatar. Your Self – capital 'S' – is the consciousness behind all of the labels and thoughts and mental chatter; the part of you which is Life itself.

Knowing that Self through direct experience – which sometimes arises spontaneously, but more commonly through practice such as meditation – is what we mean by Self-realisation.

The foundational yoga text is the Yoga Sutras of Patanjali, believed to have been written around 2500 years ago. Patanjali was a great sage – an enlightened master – who laid down the path to *samadhi* (bliss) and *kaivalya* (ultimate freedom) in this seminal text. He defines yoga right at the beginning of the Sutras as '*yogah citta vrtti nirodhah*' – 'yoga is the cessation of the fluctuations of consciousness'; or, 'yoga stills the fluctuations of the mind'.

Yoga is both the state of absolute stillness of mind, and the practices which we undertake to find that stillness. As the Sutras go on to explain, our suffering results largely from the wrestling of our minds – our misunderstandings surrounding who we really are and of situations; our misidentification with ego labels; and our attachments, aversions and insecurities. Yoga offers us a path to freedom from our suffering, and there's a twist – it's not something that can be achieved or won, because we've all had it all along. The state of blissful freedom that is yoga is our natural dwelling place – we just cover it up with myriad layers of human angst, and we forget. Yoga is a process of uncovering and revealing, rather than acquiring - a means of attaining what we already have. Yoga is the way home.

The word *yoga* means union, and yoga practices and philosophy are about bringing together the different aspects that make up a human being, creating balance in each of them so that we can live happier, more fulfilled lives. Yoga offers us a path to liberation from the stormy weather of our own minds, whilst realising our fullest potential in the world.

It's not a religion. It's not a belief system. Yoga is practical, positive, and experiential. Yoga doesn't tell you what to see, but instead takes you by the hand and invites you to come and find out for yourself.

<u>What the Sutras Say</u>

1.1 Atha yoganusasanam

1.2 Yogah citta vrtti nirodhah

1.3 Tada drastuh svarupe avasthanam

This is yoga:
Yoga stills the fluctuations of the mind,
Then you can see things as they really are.

So how does it work?

The yoga tradition says that a human being is made up of five different aspects called *koshas*, meaning layers or sheaths. We can imagine them like a Russian doll:

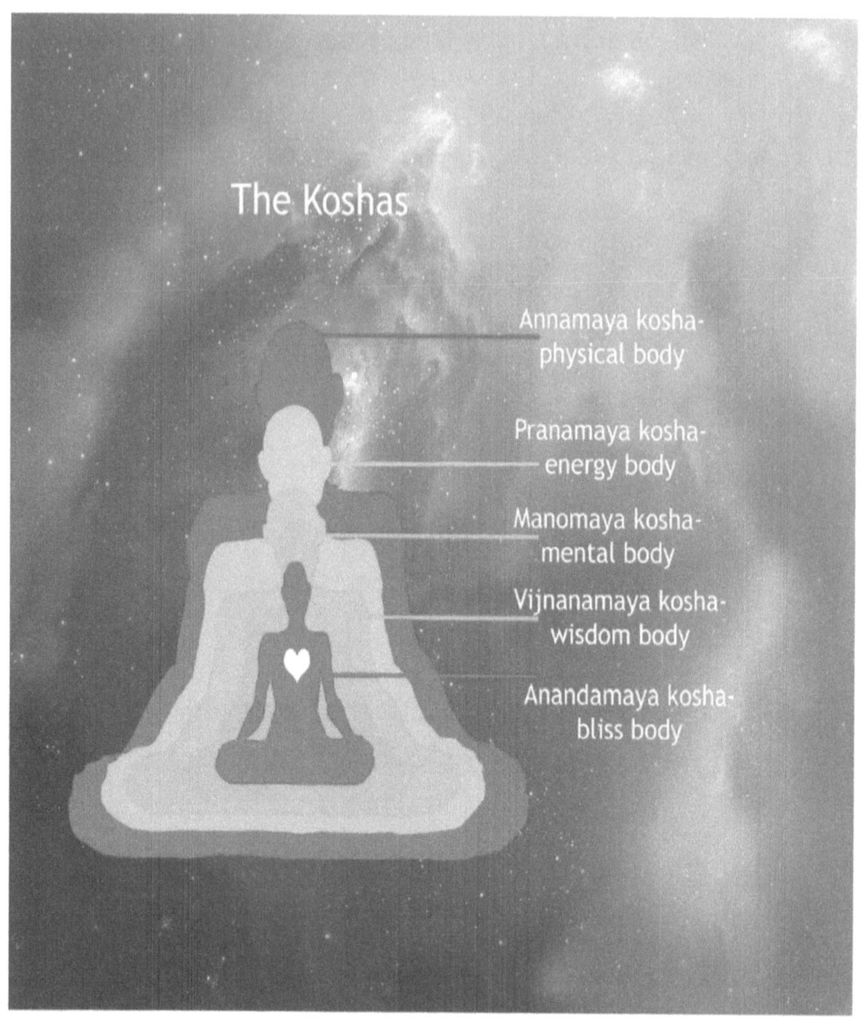

These five layers encompass and describe the whole human, and the practice of yoga works on all of them to bring us into a state of balance – it is a true 'holistic' methodology.

<u>First layer</u>

The first layer, and the one we're most familiar with, is our physical body, called **annamaya kosha**. This is our anatomy and physiology; our vehicle, our physical contact with the world, where we receive information about our surroundings, express ourselves, and perform actions in the world. The yoga postures we practise help to keep our physical bodies strong, mobile, supple and healthy; and of course our bodies also require other forms of care such as good food, fresh water, enough sleep and regular exercise.

<u>Second layer</u>

The second layer is our energy, called **pranamaya kosha**. *Prana* means energy, and the *pranamaya kosha* describes the physiological systems of the body in conjunction with *annamaya kosha*, as well as the subtle energy distribution and movements of the *nadis, chakras* and *vayus*, which we will explore in chapter 12.

You are a part of the Universe, and the Universe is a part of you. Every time you breathe in, you inhale the Universe's energy into you. Every time you exhale, you send a part of you into the universal energy. Your energy is inextricably connected with the Universe, like the atoms which make up your body. These atoms have not always been 'you' – you are quite literally made of stardust, and everything in the Universe is alive with energy. Think of the electrons in atoms. Pure energy.

We can all relate to having high or low energy levels at different times; sometimes we feel tired and lethargic, sometimes we're vibrant and raring to go. If you pause for a moment now and close your eyes, you might be able to detect this energy as a slight tingling or vibration under your skin, a sense of aliveness. You can probably also feel your heartbeat and the way your breathing subtly moves your body. This is all *prana* – the life-force. We require energy in the forms of ample oxygen from full breathing, adequate rest, and sustenance from nourishing foods such as fresh vegetables and fruit, full of vitality. Time spent doing things we love, sunlight and our human and animal interactions also give us energy – think about how full of life and nourished you feel after a great day with friends or a walk in nature; or consider how you might feel tired, then get exciting news and feel a burst of life. Now consider how some interactions leave you feeling drained. There's more going on there than the physical movement of energy in the form of glucose and oxygen – there's a felt sense of being recharged or depleted; and that's all *prana*. A rounded yoga practice helps us to regulate and direct our energy through a balance of activity and rest, and through the expanded breathing which is such a huge part of yoga's toolkit.

As a yoga practice deepens, our subtle awareness of our own energy evolves and becomes more refined, helping us to keep our 'batteries' fully charged and avoid burnout. Furthermore, we develop an awareness of the energies around us and how we are so intricately connected to the Universe. As Einstein said, 'everything in life is vibration'; and Nikola Tesla, who designed our modern AC electricity supply and invented X-ray imaging, is credited with saying: 'if you want to find the secrets of the Universe, think in terms of energy, frequency and vibration'.

Einstein knew it and Tesla knew it. The energy of the Universe is not some fairy story. This is quantum physics!

<u>Third layer</u>

The third layer is our minds and psychological state, known as **manomaya kosha**. This is where we plan, think and analyse, and also where we find our ego, desires, fears, judgements, repetitive thoughts and mental chatter. Our minds use three processes which we will investigate in this section, called *manas* (everyday thinking mind), *ahamkara* (ego) and *buddhi* (intelligence).

We often hear about 'quieting the mind', and so it's important to understand that our minds are not the enemy. They're incredible feats of biology and we'd be pretty stuck without them – we just have to learn how to put them to their best use as a kind of super-computer rather than captain of the ship. As the saying goes, 'the mind makes a great servant and a terrible master'! Through yoga practices, which refine concentration and lead us into a state of meditation, we learn how to watch our thoughts as an onlooker. We become aware of our own mental patterns, and learn to steady our runaway thinking, the better to use our mind's intelligence to help rather than hinder us. We move towards taming and reframing our less helpful, repetitive thoughts, and in this way we can literally rewire our own brains through the phenomenon of neuroplasticity, in the same way that a stroke survivor can learn to perform an action again even if the part of their brain that previously governed that action is irreparably damaged. Over time we become familiar with our own patterns, learn to recognise thoughts for what they are – passing energetic events, rather than absolute reality - and from there find a sense of peacefulness and space within our own heads.

Throughout yoga texts, the word *'citta'* appears a lot. *Citta* describes our human minds. Our everyday minds have three principle processes or parts.

Manas: This is the part of the mind which organises input from the senses and translates it to output in the form of action. *Manas* is the thinking mind and principally concerns itself with past and future events, planning and creating impressions from what it has learnt, and co-ordinating our everyday activities. This would be brilliant if we used it only as a tool, employed when there's a job for it to do and suspended at other times, but for most of us that's not how it is. *Manas* becomes the monkey mind which, when out of control, is easily distracted and torments us with constant chatter, worry and repetitive thoughts.

Ahamkara: Literally meaning 'I-maker', *ahamkara* is the ego. The ego according to the yoga tradition is a little different from how we might understand the word in western psychology. It's not so much a case of someone having a big ego and thinking they're the bee's knees, or it being a necessary part of our psychology in order to function in the world. In yoga, ego describes the roles and labels which we adopt, and how we identify ourselves. It can lead us into trouble because of its proclivity for identifying with external objects, affiliations, possessions, roles, labels and appearances. Like a house of cards, when our sense of who we are is falsely built upon impermanent structures, we are doomed to suffer when circumstances change. Statements that begin 'I am a....' are indicators of these roles and labels which we use to define ourselves. Such statements are practical in general conversation, but the trouble starts when we believe them at a deeper level. Ego has little to do with the present moment; for example, I am only a teacher when I am actually teaching. At other times I may be a walker, a driver, a gardener, a swimmer, a reader – but only for as long as I am actually engaged in that activity. In truth, when not engaged in an activity, I am simply… me. Simply being.

It's a bit like The Invisible Man, who wore clothing to make himself seen to the outside world. If our true Self is pure Consciousness, the ego is the collection of clothing which we wear to define ourselves to the outside world, and when we start to believe that self-image, we can run into difficulties and suffer when it's challenged.

Buddhi: With the same root, '*budh*', meaning 'to awaken' as the name of the Buddha, *buddhi* is our intellect and intelligence. Whilst it's more refined and less troublesome than *manas* and *ahamkara* in the normal scheme of things, and absolutely vital for us to live our lives, *buddhi* can still lead us astray. Some highly intellectual people live entirely from their analytical heads, with little intuition, felt sense of understanding, or awareness of themselves as something greater than their clever brains. These people might fool themselves into believing that they have great understanding of a subject, when in reality they have absorbed nothing of its essence – for example, someone who can chant all 196 Sutras in Sanskrit from memory and know, intellectually, what they all mean, but who hasn't truly realised any of their teachings at a deeper level. At its most refined, *buddhi* becomes richer than a purely mental process and is the difference between understanding something intellectually and really grasping it on a far deeper level – like those moments when something you have known on a surface level really lands with you and you 'get it' in an 'aha' moment.

So in the manomaya kosha we have:

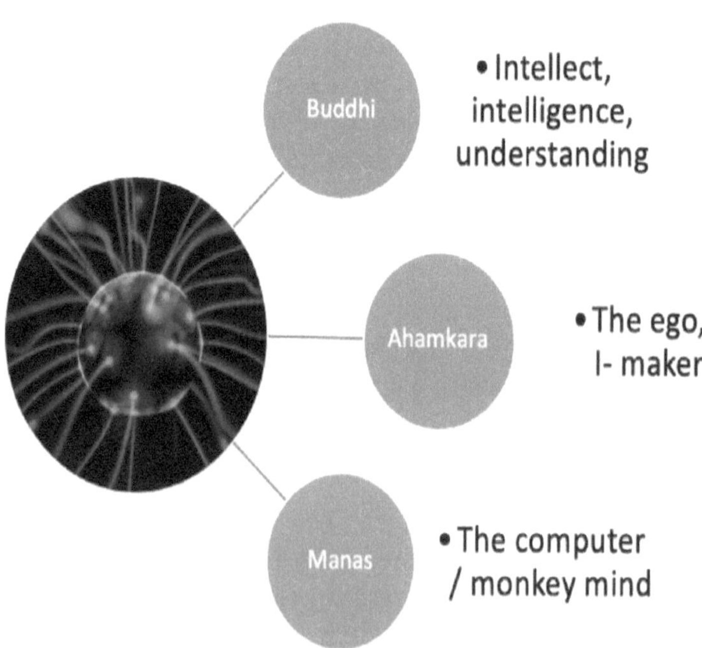

Patanjali describes the mind as having five activities (sutras 1.5 – 1.11), which can be either helpful or problematic. They are:

Pramana – correct understanding, right knowledge
Viparyaya – misapprehension, misunderstanding
Vikalpa – imagination, mental construct
Nidra – sleep
Smrtayah – memory

Yoga aims to discover and reduce the causes of misapprehension and erroneous mental constructs, in order to diminish our own suffering.

<u>Fourth layer</u>

Moving further inwards to the fourth layer, we meet **vijnanamaya kosha**. This is our intuition, wisdom, insight and inspiration; our true intelligence, beyond thought. This is where we have a quiet sense of knowing - but we don't always listen. Have you ever said 'I knew I should / shouldn't have done that'? That was your intuition – your inner teacher - trying to get your attention. When we're busy overthinking – caught up in the wrangling of an untamed *manomaya kosha* – it can be almost impossible to access this quietly-knowing part of ourselves. When we practice steadying the mind, as our concentration improves and our meditation practice deepens, our ability to connect with our own inner guidance is enhanced because we can recognise our brain chatter for what it is, and we learn to hear beyond the noise to our quieter inner wisdom. With practice, we experience greater clarity and intuitive insight, and learn to trust ourselves.

<u>Fifth layer</u>

The subtlest aspect of a human, called **anandamaya kosha**, translates as 'blissful joy body'. We fleetingly experience this joy-filled part of ourselves when when we are completely present or 'in flow' and time seems to stop; there is no mental commentary, no value judgement, just complete engagement with the moment. Different things take us to our blissful place - nature, dancing, music, playing with an animal, deep connection with a loved one. (Joy – *ananda* - is distinct from pleasure – *kama* - and whilst there's nothing wrong with pleasure, it's different from pure joy. It's interesting to notice that our experiences of true joy tend to be both free and non-harmful!)

These subtler *koshas* of *vijnanamaya* and *anandamaya* – intuition and bliss – bring us closer to our true nature of pure Consciousness, the flame which is sheathed by the *koshas*. Ultimately yoga liberates us, little by little, from the torments of our minds and self-created dramas, and we experience this state more and more. Enlightenment is the state of existing in this internal yet expanded environment of non-attached awareness at all times – not something that is likely for most of us! - but regular yoga practice equips us to experience this part of ourselves on a more frequent basis; to connect with our own unique purpose or *dharma* (see chapter 16); and to live happier, more fulfilled lives.

But... HOW?

The secret that yoga unlocks for us is this: these subtler layers such as intuition and bliss are not an external thing that can be acquired, because they already exist inside of us. Yoga is a process of stripping away the additional layers of behaviours, reactions and learned responses that we accumulate as we go through life; it helps us to see things as they really are. That peaceful, still, joyous refuge inside us is always there, but life gets in the way and we forget our true nature. Yoga shows us how to remember, and gives us access to our own constant 'yoga retreat' inside ourselves. As we'll explore throughout this book, there is a great deal more to yoga than the postures (*asanas*) – it is nothing less than a complete system for living our best possible lives.

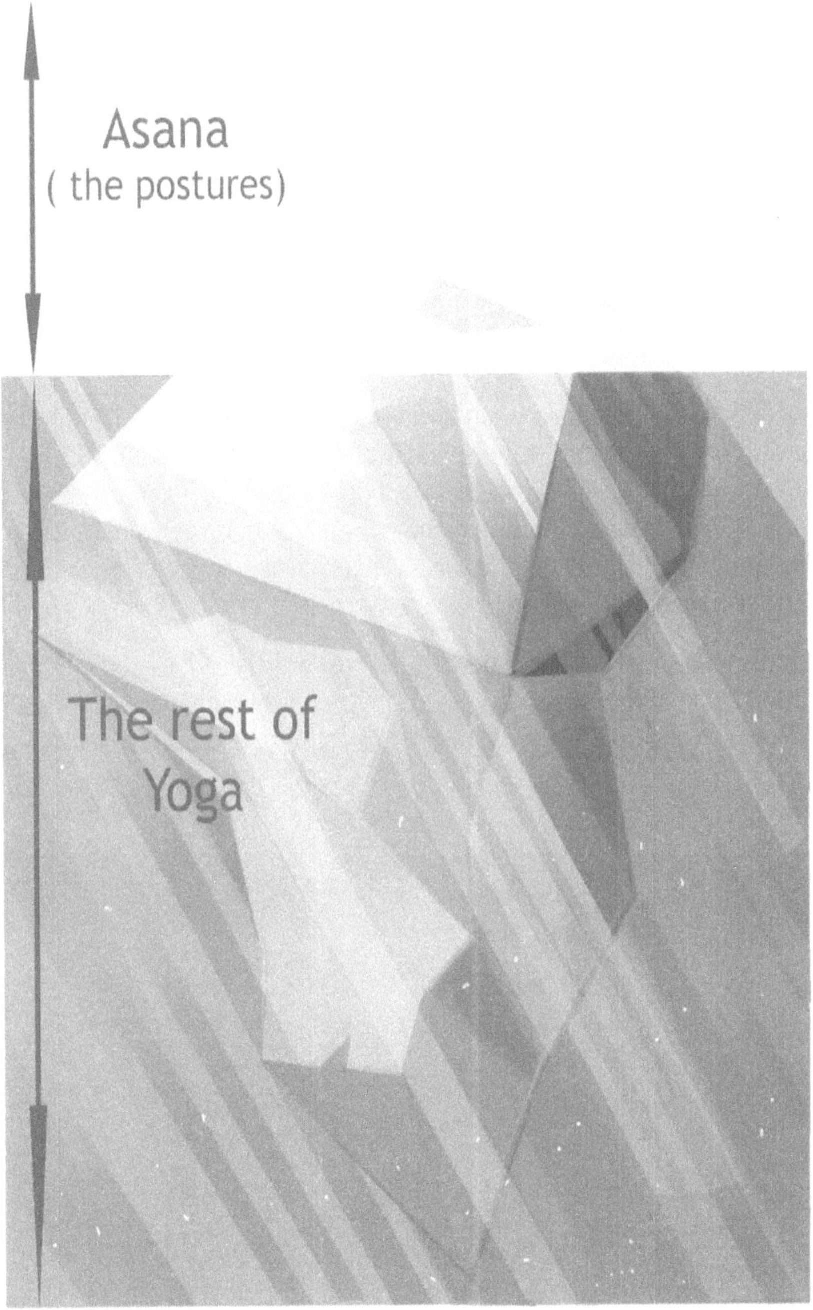

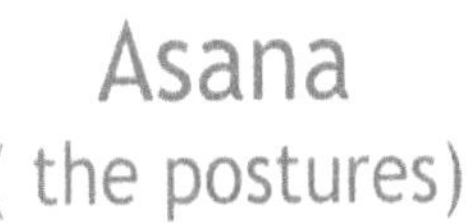

Asana
(the postures)

The rest of
Yoga

Chapter 2 – An Introduction to the Eight Limbs of Yoga

The previous chapter illustrated the different parts of what constitutes a human according to the yoga tradition. Now let's look at how yoga can bring those parts into harmony with the world.

The *Yoga Sutras* are a step by step treatise on the philosophy of yoga by the great sage Patanjali consisting of 196 brief aphorisms divided across four chapters. '*Sutra*' means thread.

Although the *Sutras* can seem mysterious and daunting at first, they form the crucial basis of the yoga that we practise today. Whilst some of the verses may seem esoteric, and anyone who is not a Sanskrit scholar will certainly need an accompanying translation and explanation, they contain a wealth of solid, profound information which is fundamental to yoga practice and absolutely relevant to modern life.

A cornerstone of yoga - and probably the most well-known teaching from the *Sutras* - is the Eight Limbs of Yoga, which we meet in the second '*pada*' or chapter (2:30). These eight areas are foundational to a well-rounded yoga practice.

The Eight Limbs of Yoga

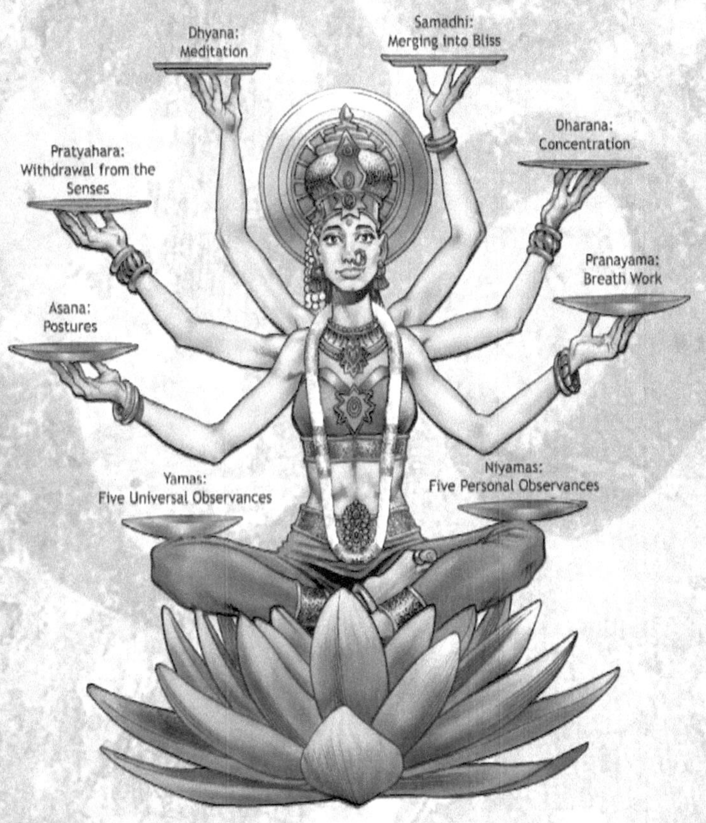

1 - *Yamas* (universal observances)
2 - *Niyamas* (personal observances)
3 - *Asana* (postures)
4 - *Pranayama* (breathwork)
5 - *Pratyahara* (withdrawal from the senses)
6 - *Dharana* (concentration)
7 - *Dhyana* (meditation)
8 - *Samadhi* (merging into bliss)

The first two limbs, the *yamas* and *niyamas*, consist of ten ethical precepts for living in harmony with ourselves, other beings, and the world around us. If we did nothing more than follow these behaviours and restraints, we would guarantee ourselves a far happier and more balanced life and we would be practising yoga. Indeed, if we all adopted the *yamas* and *niyamas*, then world peace and a healthy planet could become a reality! Imagine a world in we which we all practised non-violence; honesty; non-stealing; appropriate use of energy; non-grasping; cleanliness; contentment; self-enquiry; enthusiastic discipline; and peaceful acceptance of the unity of Life as the bond which unites us all! The *yamas* and *niyamas* are a framework for greater self-awareness, to lead us to greater happiness.

The limbs of *asana* (postures) and *pranayama* (breathwork) are the aspects of yoga with which we are generally most familiar, as they are the ones most widely taught in classes.

The limbs become more subtle as we continue on, and one limb tends to lead to the next as we refine our practice: for example, when we combine *asana* with *pranayama* we find our attention directed inwards, away from the distractions of the outside world (*pratyahara*). Concentration (*dharana*) prepares us to enter a state of meditation (*dhyana*). Eventually, after much practice, we may experience and then reside in a state of bliss (*samadhi*) as we merge into a felt-sense of unity with the Universe. Whilst the eight limbs are typically described sequentially and separately for the sake of clarity, in reality they are all interwoven.

Whilst many contemporary yoga classes place a lot of emphasis on *asana*, the physical postures are just a fraction of what is on offer in the vast world of yoga, much of which will be explored throughout this book.

Together, the eight limbs of yoga form a framework for a fully integrated, higher way of living. Like an adventure guidebook, they show us the way to explore the different aspects of being human, fine-tune our subtle awareness, and enable us to experience a richer, more fulfilling life.

Over the coming chapters, we'll look at each limb in depth, and explore its relevance to our modern everyday lives.

The Eight Limbs of Yoga

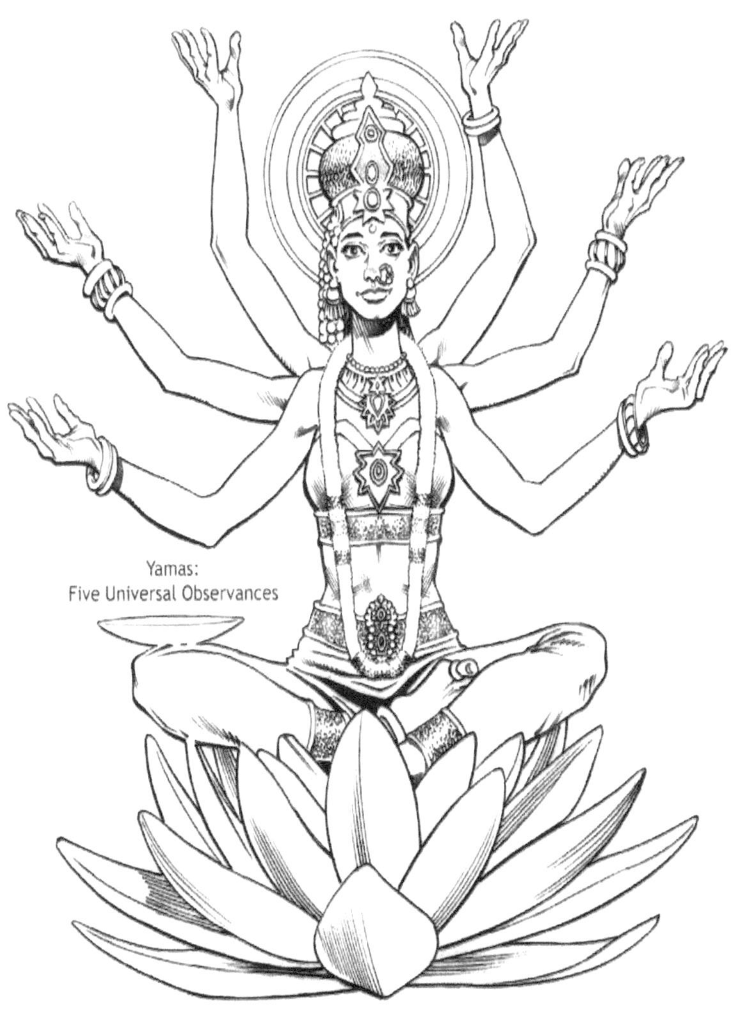

Ahimsa or non-violence
Satya or truthfulness

Asteya or non-stealing
Brahmacharya or continence / appropriate use of energy
Aparigraha or non-grasping / letting go

The *yamas* are general guidelines for wise living. They might seem like obvious values at first glance, but take a closer look and they become more nuanced. Yoga is all about fine-tuning your subtle awareness, and applying the *yamas* to everyday life is a wonderful way to really start to live your yoga.

<u>*Ahimsa*: Non-violence; peacefulness</u>

Ahimsa - non-violence - is the first universal principle of yoga. Cultivating a peaceful attitude towards all beings and to our planet is the first step to higher, integrated living, and the path towards making our own life and the world at large a better place to be.

Whilst it's pretty obvious that killing or being physically violent is a bad thing, there are far subtler ways in which we inflict violence. *Ahimsa* begins with our attitude towards ourselves. When we offer compassion to ourselves, as we would to a friend or loved one, rather than beating ourselves up for some perceived shortcoming, we are practising *ahimsa*. When we take care of our bodies by nourishing them with fresh, healthy food and exercise, rather than filling them with junk and not moving enough, we are practising *ahimsa*. When we make sure that we get adequate sleep and downtime, rather than staying up too late and pushing ourselves into burnout, we are practising *ahimsa*. It's all about non-harming; offering compassion to ourselves and all things; not making things worse and perhaps making them a tiny bit better. The renowned teacher David Swenson has a lovely interpretation of 'what makes a yogi'. He says that 'a yogi leaves a place a little nicer than they found it'. So how else can we bring this idea into daily life? There are myriad ways, but here are some suggestions to get you started - try them on for size, add your own, and see if you can maintain a background awareness of *ahimsa*.

- In your yoga class, offer your body appreciation for what it CAN do, rather than comparing it with the super-bendy person next to you. So they have very open hips - it doesn't make them a better person! Don't push or force your body beyond where it wants to go - sensation is fine, pain never is. Your amazing body carries you around all day and lets you experience life, so give it some love and recognition. After all, where else are you going to live?

- Leave an environment (your bedroom, the office, nature) at least as nice as you found it. Clear up after yourself, and if you can see something else (a coffee cup, a bit of litter) that wasn't your mess, that you could deal with in seconds, do that too.

- Choose nourishing food that your body (not just your taste-buds or your emotions!) wants. Imagining your internal organs can make you think twice when tempted by unhealthy snacks.

- *Ahimsa* is often interpreted as necessitating a diet free from animal produce, and certainly animal agriculture is having a devastating impact on our planet's resources and inevitably involves the killing and exploitation of other beings. Switching to a plant-powered way of life is a personal choice that many find themselves naturally gravitating towards with a yogic lifestyle, but if we do choose to eat meat, fish, dairy and eggs, we can buy less but buy better. Organically reared meat and dairy animals have slightly higher standards of care; responsibly sourced fish rather than trawled means we do less damage to our precious oceans; and replacing as much as possible of our animal-based intake with plant-based foods means a vastly reduced impact on the planet's resources.

- Words can hurt or heal, so think before you speak. Ask yourself: 'Is it true? Is it kind? Is it necessary?'

- Be kind, even when someone is being unkind. *Especially* when someone is being unkind. We don't know what goes on in other people's lives, so try to reserve judgment - they might be having an awful time in their personal lives and you just happened to be in the line of fire. That doesn't mean being a doormat - if you're being treated unfairly, of course you should stand up for yourself - that's *ahimsa* too. But there's always a way to do that without attacking the other person - it can be as simple as saying, 'this is not ok' or 'I'm not willing to be spoken to in that way', or 'when you do *x*, I feel as though *y* - could we find a time to talk about this please?'

Those are just a few ideas – there are many many more. We can all make our shared world a better place to be by practising *ahimsa*. It's a fantastic way to start bringing the deeper aspects of yoga into your everyday life - just imagine a world in which everyone practised *ahimsa*! It starts with each and every one of us, in each and every moment.

As the Dalai Lama says: 'Be kind whenever possible. It's **always** possible.'

<u>*Satya*: Honesty; truthfulness</u>

Satya means truthfulness. Seems pretty obvious, right? But like its forerunner *ahimsa*, if we dig a little deeper we discover a wealth of hidden meanings within this simple concept.

Like *ahimsa*, the practice of *satya* begins with ourselves - it's difficult to make progress in any endeavour without first honestly acknowledging where we really are. This applies to all aspects of life - if we want to improve our financial situation, we first need to take an honest look at our debts and spending habits. If we want to enhance our relationships, we have to acknowledge what we bring to the table, both the helpful and the challenging. If we want to develop our fitness levels, it's no use kidding ourselves that the gym membership alone will do it - we have to actually go!

But if it's brashly handled, honesty can cause pain, and so it has to be balanced with non-violence. An elderly relative suffering from dementia may believe that they are in their youth and surrounded by childhood friends, family and pets. Is there any kindness in reminding them that they are actually in a nursing home? Just because something is true, doesn't mean it's always appropriate to shove the facts in someone's face. Again, asking ourselves 'Is it true? Is it kind? Is it necessary?' is a good litmus test for when to speak out and when to remain silent, and so practise compassionate, benevolent honesty. This distinction is called *rtyam* and *satyam* – where *satyam* is the whole, unadulterated truth, and *rtyam* is appropriate truth. When we develop our *viveka* or wise discernment, we learn how to apply discretion.

How else might we apply *satya* to everyday life?

- On the yoga mat, by honouring where our bodies are today and not pushing beyond our limits, and by maintaining appropriate alignment for our own body's structure rather than compromising the safe benefits of the pose for a flashy demonstration.

- By being realistic about how much time is needed to complete a task, so we don't overstress ourselves.

- By acknowledging difficult feelings, rather than muscling past them. It's ok to feel doubtful, scared, angry, depressed, anxious, jealous, frustrated - we're human. Until we acknowledge what's really going on, we can't begin to address it and find ways to process and move on. It's incredible how much power simply acknowledging feelings has to loosen their grip on us.

- By saying 'no' when we need to. If you're an over-explainer, and feel that you have to give a lengthy (and possibly untrue) excuse as to why you're turning down a request or invitation, try having a few phrases up your sleeve, such as: 'Thank you, but I have other plans'; 'I'm afraid that won't be convenient'; or 'I appreciate the offer, but I'm not taking anything else on right now'. It feels really good to honour our own healthy boundaries - and never lying means never having to remember what we've said to whom!

- By being true to ourselves in the way we live. Life is short - why follow someone else's script? Be guided by your intuition and write your own story that feels authentic to *you*.

But the deepest level of *satya* lies at the very heart of yoga. The word *sat* comes up a lot in the Sanskrit texts and it means 'the true essence, that which is unchangeable'; far more than simply 'truth' as in 'not lying'. The purpose of yoga practice is to learn to quieten the mind, to peel back the layers and gradually glimpse the essence of our being - the True Self - the enduring presence within. Every time you come to the mat or meditation cushion, every time you live your yoga, you engage in this process and your practice matures a little. As Krishna says to Arjuna in the *Bhagavad Gita*: 'No effort on this path is wasted, no gain is ever reversed; even a little of this practice will shelter you from the greatest sorrow'.

Asteya: Non-stealing

Just like the previous two *yamas*, *asteya* or non-stealing seems pretty self-explanatory - we don't go round taking other people's belongings, and we've known that since childhood. But in common with its predecessors, there's more to practising *asteya* than meets the eye.

Do you find your mind or eyes wandering when someone's talking to you?

Do you dismiss compliments paid to you? Do you find yourself staying up later than you'd intended - watching TV or just messing about - when you'd promised yourself an early night? Each of these is an example of how we might subtly steal from ourselves and others. When we allow ourselves to be distracted during a conversation, we rob both ourselves and our companions of the opportunity for real connection. When we dismiss a compliment rather than simply saying 'thank you', we rob the giver of their attempt to make us feel appreciated. And when we allow our good habits to fall by the wayside, we rob ourselves not only of those health benefits, but also of the feeling of being proud of ourselves for practising self-care.

So how do we practise *asteya*? When we become aware of these tiny, insidious acts, we can make the conscious choice to do the opposite, and explore how that might feel instead. The opposite of stealth-stealing is a generosity of spirit, both to ourselves and others. Here are some of the ways in which we might steal without realising it - try observing your own behaviour and exploring opportunities to practise *asteya*.

- Placing our own expectations on others. When we label our partner 'the strong one', we rob them of the chance to show us their vulnerability, as well as robbing ourselves of the chance to truly know them behind the mask we've imposed upon them. When we try too hard to steer a child down a certain route because they show an aptitude, we rob them of the chance to express themselves as they wish. When we fail to see our parents as human beings with private lives and feelings, we all miss out on the chance for a greater understanding of each other.

- Poking around in someone else's belongings, such as rifling through our partner's bedside drawer when they're out, or reading a friend's journal when you house-sit for them, is stealing their privacy.

- Giving unsolicited advice is a way of subtly stealing a person's capacity to solve their own problems.

- Parking inconsiderately, such as spanning two spaces rather than getting close enough to the next car, is stealing a space (and therefore time and convenience) from the next person who comes along.

- Hiding our light under a bushel. None of us are special, but every one of us is unique, and we each have talents which can benefit others. False modesty and shyness deprive the world of your gifts and serve no-one.

- Guilt-trips. There's no point indulging yourself once in a while if you're going to steal all the fun away by going on a guilt-trip afterwards. If you're going to do it, do it: eat the piece of cake / watch the trashy TV show / treat yourself to the dress - and OWN your decision and your pleasure. As long as it's occasional and you're not damaging yourself or others, aren't life's frivolous little treats to be savoured and enjoyed?

- Poor time-keeping. If you're teaching a yoga class, it might seem generous to overrun and give students an extra ten minutes of your time, but we never know people's circumstances. They might be on a tight schedule, have a baby-sitter they promised they'd be home for, or have to catch a particular train – so the teacher's misplaced generosity actually has a knock-on effect and steals from the rest of their day.

- Taking the easy road. If we always stay in our comfort zones and never challenge ourselves, we rob ourselves of the chance to discover what we're really capable of; and it's usually way more than we think.

- Cancelling plans at the last minute or being late. We don't know what other commitments people might have moved around in order to spend time with us, and lateness and last-minute cancellations, (unless the circumstances are exceptional) effectively signal that the other person's time is less important than our own – which is a form of stealing.

How else can you imagine that you might stealth-steal from yourself and others? There are many ways in which we subtly undermine others and steal their joy, peace of mind, and so on. How might you turn that around and practise *asteya* instead?

<u>*Brahmacharya*: Continence; appropriate use of energy</u>

Brahmacharya is a little trickier to define in western terms than its predecessors. Its direct translation is 'merging into one-ness with the Divine', but what does that actually mean? Broadly speaking, it's to do with how we use our energy and maintaining healthy boundaries. More specifically it refers to sexual energy, and how we choose to share our sexuality. Some ancient yogi ascetics took it to its limits and practised celibacy, but for those of us who don't live in isolation, meditating for years in caves in the

Himalayas, it's a little more fluid. For 'householder yogis' like you and me, the sexual aspect of *brahmacharya* is to do with healthy, mutually respectful intimate relationships, and refraining from using our sexual energy in ways likely to cause suffering either to ourselves or others. It's a tricky subject because we all have our own ideas of what consitutes acceptable sexual behaviour. Are casual hook-ups ok? Do we wait until the third date? Until we're engaged? Married?

The tenets of yoga are intended as guidelines, and they invite – and are robust enough to stand up to - intelligent self-enquiry. So whilst it's wholly up to the individual how they conduct their intimate life, contemplating *brahmacharya* offers a wise framework for intimate relationships. We might ask ourselves questions like:

- Is everyone in this liaison being treated with compassion and respect?

- Does everyone understand where they stand? Are they on the same page, or is one party in it for the long-haul and the other playing the field?

- Are all parties being open and honest with each other?

- Is everyone happy and fulfilled within the situation, or is someone being coerced into behaving in a way they're not comfortable with?

- If there is a mutual expectation of monogamy, is it being honoured? Do both parties feel secure and confident of the other's fidelity?

- Are both parties honoured as the only one, or is there a habit of commenting on attractive third parties?

Our sexual energy, shared wisely, can be one of the most life-affirming parts of our human experience - something to be revered and celebrated. Sex between partners with a true connection can be a deeply spiritual experience, when our barriers dissolve and we merge into one-ness - the literal definition of *brahmacharya* - together.

Whilst sexuality is the central theme of this yama, an additional interpretation encompasses our boundaries in other parts of our lives - how we use our energy in a wider sense. If you regularly find yourself saying 'yes' to things that you don't really want to do in order to please other people; if you're overwhelmed and never have time for yourself because of demands that you routinely give in to; if you don't feel that your needs are as important as everyone else's; if you find it hard to keep information given in confidence to yourself; if you feel that your rights to be heard, express yourself freely, and not be touched without permission are not respected; then it might be time to reassess the boundaries that you set, and become more assertive in maintaining them. People with healthy boundaries generally also have healthy levels of self-respect and self-esteem. They are firm but flexible, asking for support when they need it, and are respectful of other people's boundaries as well as maintaining their own. They understand that they are responsible for themselves and their own wellbeing. They are compassionate with others but are clear about what belongs to them, listening fully and being helpful but not taking on other people's problems. They understand what they need in order to feel supported and respected, and are confident about making sure they receive it.

When we practise *brahmacharya*, the people around us feel valued, secure and confident that they can trust us to treat them with kindness and respect. And, importantly, we feel that way about ourselves!

Aparigraha: Non-grasping; letting go

The fifth and final *yama* is *aparigraha*, or non-grasping / non-attachment; and letting go.

Some examples of grasping behaviours are jealousy at another's success; bitterness when someone has material possessions, talents or relationships which we covet; taking more than is freely offered; and becoming attached to expectations and outcomes.

Grasping is closely tied up with greed, jealousy, and control, all of which arise from a sense of not being enough or having enough. In its most extreme expression, grasping can take the form of hoarding, stalking, and trying to control others.

Of course most of us never go that far, but a touch of grasping is a very common thing. We get attached to the idea of how a holiday is going to be - and then come crashing down with disappointment when it falls short. We take more food than we really need - and then feel over-stuffed and guilty. We experience retail-lust and have to have the shiny new bauble - then avoid opening our bank statements. We feel jealous of a friend's seemingly perfect relationship with their partner – but know little of the couple's private struggles. And of course, in these days of social media, we compare ourselves with idealised images of beautiful people in dream locations - and inevitably find ourselves failing to measure up.

If only we realised just how little we need, how perfect we are just the way we are, and how much the world needs our unique expressions of ourselves. If only we realised that expectation will almost always be better than reality, and that comparison is the thief of joy. If only we could relax and enjoy what's in front of us, without measuring it up against an imagined ideal. If only we realised that we already have what we need, right here inside us.

The realisation that we have all we need, and that it's all around us, is called living in abundance. Feeling gratitude for the things which we ordinarily take for granted is a simple but profound practice and an effective means of tasting *aparigraha*. Living with a sense of abundance and gratitude means that we rarely feel poor, or jealous, or bitter, because gratitude turns what we have into enough. When we regularly focus on all that we are grateful for, it matters less what someone else has, and we realise how full of reasons to be happy our own lives are. When we come from a mindset of abundance - that we have enough and *are* enough, it takes greed out at the knees.

Keeping a gratitude journal is a fantastic way to get started in culitivating *aparigraha*. Each day, write down three things which you're grateful for. There are plenty - you're reading this, so you have a level of education, functioning eyesight and the freedom to read what you choose.

I'm guessing that you didn't sleep in the street last night, that you have access to safe drinking water and sanitation, and that you know where your next meal is coming from. What else? Are you healthy? Do you live in a relatively safe country? Is there someone in your life who you love? There are so many things to be grateful for when we look, and the lovely thing is that once you start becoming aware of them the effect snowballs.

There's nothing wrong with enjoying nice things and wanting life's comforts, just as long as we don't become so attached to them that we suffer when they're not around or feel painfully jealous when someone else has what we want. There's nothing wrong with making plenty of money doing something you're good at – money is just a form of energy, and when we have more of it we can help more people. There's nothing wrong with admiring others and finding inspiration in them, as long as we don't get caught up in comparison and lose ourselves in the process. It's all about becoming aware of how much we already have and celebrating that. And when we generously celebrate the good fortune of others too, and feel happy for them, then we get to multiply the joy we experience many times over.

There is enough to go around. A candle flame which lights another candle is in no way diminished by sharing its light. That single tiny flame can light a million other flames and never suffer from the process.

Non-grasping is knowing that you have enough, and that you are enough.

Non-attachment is the art of holding things lightly, of not clinging to experiences, possessions, people, situations, identities and so on. 'Let it go' has been used and abused to the point of becoming a cliché, but beneath the bumper sticker new-age fluff lies a profound wisdom which appears in other guises throughout the Yoga Sutras. Happiness, we are told in sutra 1.12, is the result of action without attachment to outcome. Sutra 2.3 outlines the main causes of suffering, the *kleshas*, one of which is *raga*, or attachment.

We suffer when things don't go our way because we're attached to our expectations.

We suffer when we don't get what we want because we're attached to an idea of how having something will be.

We suffer when we DO get what we want, because then we fear losing it.

Non-attachment is not the same as detachment. Non-attachment means wholeheartedly enjoying what is in front of us right now, in full acceptance of the impermanence of all things and without clinging on. Detachment implies hardening ourselves and not letting ourselves get too close to anything or anyone for fear of loss, whereas non-attachment is a radical acceptance of the inevitability of loss and impermanence, and living wholeheartedly anyway.

These five *yamas* – universal observances – are all about how we relate to others and conduct ourselves in the world. As guidelines for ethical and honourable living, they give us a reference point to come back to when we're stuck with a decision or confused about how to proceed. They keep us acting respectfully from the very best part of ourselves - if we're upholding the values of non-violence (*ahimsa*), honesty (*satya*), non-stealing (*asteya*), continence (*brahmacharya*), and non-grasping (*aparigraha*), we're unlikely to go too far wrong in our relationships and interactions in the wider world.

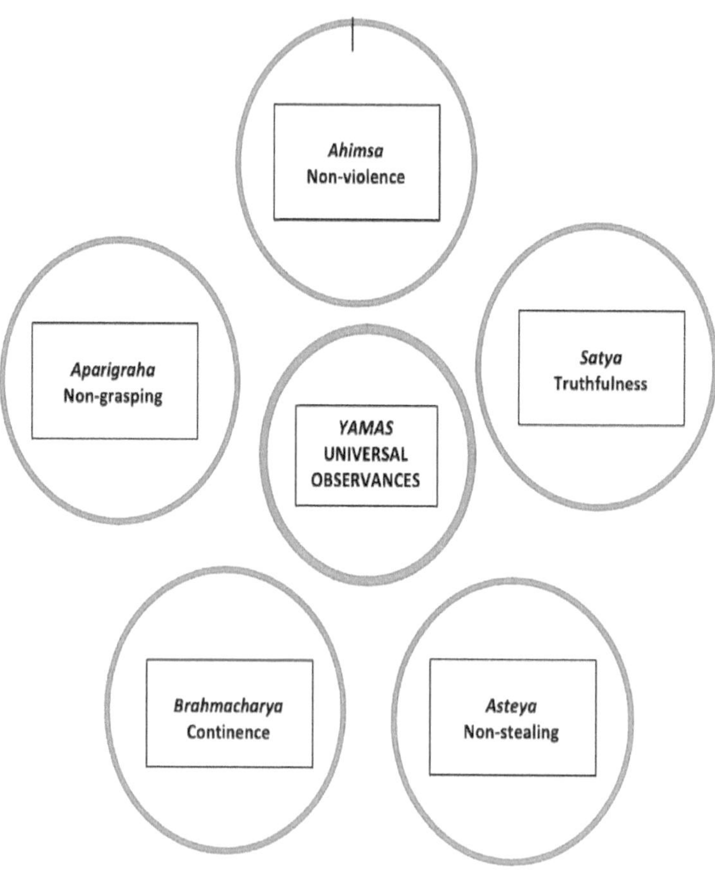

The Eight Limbs of Yoga

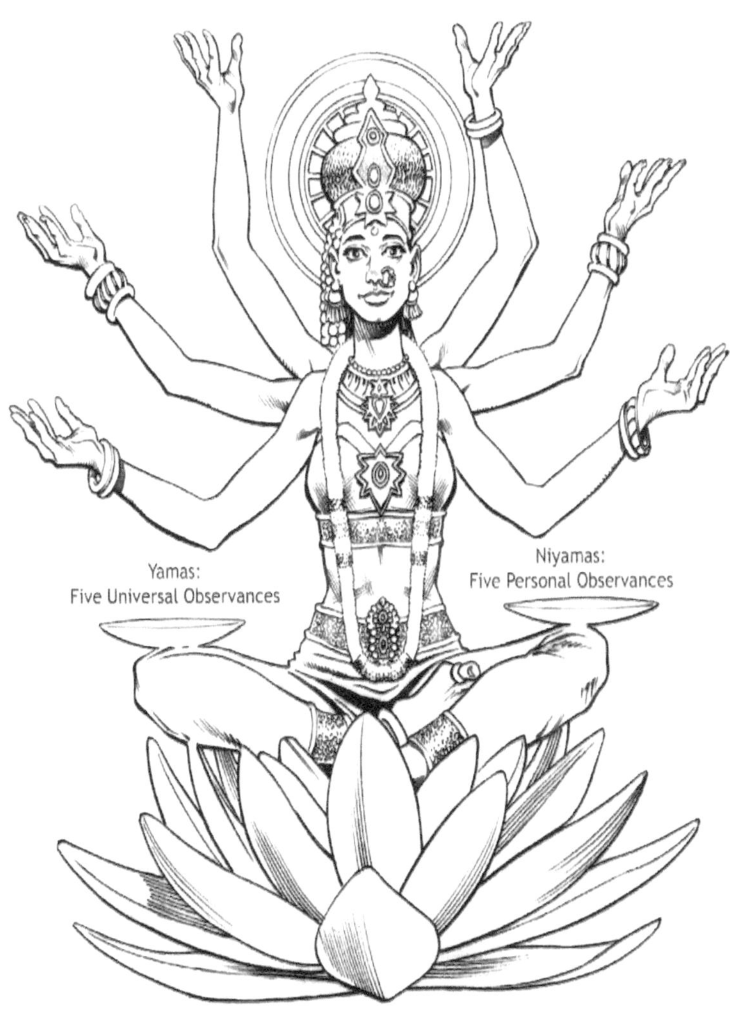

Saucha or Cleanliness
Santosha or Contentment

Svadhyaya or Self-study
Tapas or Discipline
Ishvara Pranidhana or Surrender

If the *yamas* are universal guidelines, the *niyamas* are more personal. Moving, as ever in yoga, from the most obvious to the most subtle, these are attitudes and behaviours to cultivate within ourselves. Their integration into our everyday lives leads to ever greater levels of personal freedom as we uncover the inner wisdom which gives us the confidence to be true to ourselves.

<u>*Saucha*: Cleanliness</u>

The idea of *saucha* is to provide a suitable dwelling-place for the *purusha*, or pure Consciousness, during our time in this body. As the renowned teacher BKS Iyengar put it: 'with cleanliness the body becomes the temple of the seer and feels the joy of self-awareness.'

One of the obstacles to being in a state of yoga is illness (sutra 1.30, see chapter 15), and so to avoid becoming unwell it's important that we maintain a healthy body, free from impurities.

We've all heard the expression 'my body is a temple' - usually used with some irony in western society - and this *niyama* may be where the phrase originated. The yoga *kriyas* which we'll meet in chapter 11, also known as the *shatkarma* or six actions, , are techniques which ancient Hatha yogis used to cleanse the body both inside and out, and these were offered as a way for the householder yogi (ie not an ascetic renunciant who lived in a Himalyan cave, but someone who lived a more convential life in scoiety) to work towards inner and outer cleanliness. Whilst some of them are still found today, such as *neti* pots for cleansing the nostrils (which some people find useful for managing allergies), others such as swallowing a length of fabric into the stomach and regurgitating it are rarely taught.

It doesn't stop at the body. Cleanliness in our external environment and surroundings help us to maintain health, clarity, and a sense of wellbeing.

So without going to extremes, how can we maintain a clean vessel for our inner light?

- Daily rituals of cleanliness such as showering, maintaining good dental hygiene, and caring for your nails and hair.

- Drinking a large glass of room temperature water on rising both rehydrates the body after 8 hours without liquid, and stimulates peristalsis, the wave-like motion of the gut, to get elimination moving.

- Eating a diet around delicious fresh vegetables and fruits, choosing organic if possible to avoid chemical pesticides.

- Avoiding known toxins such as nicotine, alcohol and drugs.

- Some schools of yoga advocate castor oil baths every Saturday. This involves pouring castor oil over your head and massaging it into your scalp, then continuing to massage your whole body with it before lying in *Savasana* for 15 minutes, then showering it off with soap. Castor oil is pretty messy, but a nice alternative is to make your own body scrub from an oil - (almond, olive or coconut are all great, or investigate what works well for your *dosha* for an *ayurvedic* (see chapter 19) option - and coarse salt or sugar.

- Unused, unloved items create a feeling of 'stuckness' around the home – like energy traps. If that sounds familiar, try the 30 day decluttering challenge. Put a big bag or basket somewhere central. On the first day you throw one item you are happy to part with into the basket, on the second day two items and so on. On day 30 you take them to charity, sell them, or give them to a good home. If you complete the challenge you'll have freed your home of 465 pieces of clutter! Creating order in our home and work environments reduces stress and brings a greater sense of clarity into our lives. Making our little corners of the world feel sanctuary-like is an important element of healthy self-care and self-respect.

- Does your diary need a cleanse? If you can't see any decent-sized gaps, how about making a commitment to honour what you've already agreed to, then consciously mark out some sacred 'nothing-time' in your diary going forward.

- Be impeccable in your speech. Say what you mean and mean what you say… but before you speak, make sure you can say yes to those crucial three questions: Is it true? Is it kind? Is it necessary?

- Start becoming more aware of your internal dialogue. Are there repetitive thoughts that go round in a loop? Try journalling about them and see if you can figure out where they're coming from. Do you frequently think 'I must remember to do x'? Get a pad of paper and have a fresh sheet each day to note down what your brain is trying to help you with. When it's on paper, you subconsciously relax a little knowing it won't get forgotten, which makes for a quieter and more spacious mind.

By honouring the principle of *saucha* in everyday life, we can clear the path of clutter and obstacles, whether mental, emotional, physical or environmental, the better to feel calm and see clearly.

Santosha: Contentment

What does contentment mean to you? Perhaps lying on a beautiful beach whilst gazing out at the ocean, sipping on a fresh coconut, dozing in the sunshine?

Whilst this sounds great, true contentment or *santosha* is not dependent on external circumstances. *Santosha* in everyday life means being able to keep your sense of peace and equanimity even when your situation is very far from ideal.

In common with *aparigraha*, one of the greatest practices to help cultivate *santosha* is gratitude. Becoming more aware of the small joys and pleasures in life means that our days, however taxing, can be sprinkled with magic. Simply paying attention to what's going on *outside* of your head, rather than *in* it, opens up whole new levels of appreciation for everyday life. Savouring your coffee rather than gulping it down and barely even noticing the flavour; focusing on the glorious sound of early morning birdsong rather than the roar of traffic beneath it; relishing the soft touch of a favourite pair of socks rather than shoving them on mindlessly; the day is full of experiences to enjoy, if we can just get out of our heads and pay attention.

Even when life is frustrating, we can flip our perspective - *pratipaksha bhavanam* - and find the kernel of goodness in our experience. Builders drilling outside your window? Not everyone has the ability to hear that. Overstuffed email inbox? You have access to a computer and you can read, write and type. Being jostled and shoved on a packed train? You are physically independent enough to be on that train in the first place.

We also become more contented when we focus on bringing value to our human relationships and interactions. When we stop what we're doing and give someone our full attention when they enter the room, we not only make *them* feel valued, but also build relationships, which are vital to our sense of connection and wellbeing. And this applies to everyone you interact with, from partners and parents and children, to petrol station checkout staff and strangers you pass on the street. Simply making eye contact and smiling says 'I see you', and fosters a greater sense of communion with other people and the world around us.

When we take the time to fully engage with our environment and feel grateful for the myriad blessings that we have, a shift starts to take place. We start to feel that life is abundant; rich with joy and opportunity. Discontentment always comes from a place of lack; a sense that whatever we have, it's not quite enough. When our perspective changes to one of abundance, our sense of satisfaction with life grows and blossoms, and we begin to embody the beautiful *niyama* of *santosha*: contentment.

Tapas: The refining fire of discipline

The third *niyama*, *tapas*, means not a selection of delicious Spanish dishes, but a burning enthusiasm and willingness to persevere. Yoga is not something that is done to us, or for us – it requires that we step up and take responsibility for our own progression, and that requires a certain amount of self-motivation. There are no gold stars or achievement medals in yoga – our progress is measured by our own inner experience and by how we relate to the world. With no framework such as the belts of karate to motivate us, we must cultivate the inner discipline to keep showing up for practice, again and again, with no promise of recognition or reward. So why do it? Because that *tapas*, that ability to show up and practice even when we don't feel like it, becomes its own reward as we feel a growing sense of wholeness, peace, and vitality. And so when we get up in the morning and don't feel like sitting in meditation, we might only sit for five minutes, but we sit anyway. When we feel low in energy and we'd rather lie on the sofa than get on the mat, we might honour that low energy and practise a restorative form of *asana*, but we get on the mat anyway. And gradually we realise that we never regret that decision; that we never show up, do our practice and then say 'I wish I hadn't done that.'

Svadhyaya: Self-enquiry; self-discovery

The fourth niyama is _svadhyaya_, or self-enquiry. This is a particularly interesting principle, because really the whole of yoga is a practice of _svadhyaya_. Every time we sit in meditation, step onto the mat, use _pranayama_, chant, commit to a _sankalpa_ or any of the many other practical aspects of a rounded practice, we enter a laboratory of self-study which invites us on a journey of the self, through the self, to the Self.

And it's this distinction between small 's' self and capital 'S' Self which lies at the heart of yoga. Learning to distinguish between the small self of our ego-mind, and the large Self which unites us with the Universe, is the jewel of practice. _Svadhyaya_ is the way to become ever more familiar with our own mental afflictions (_kleshas_ – see chapter 14_)_ and learned behaviours (_samskaras_ – see chapter 15_)_, the better to see life more clearly.

This practice of self-enquiry is ripe for weaving through our everyday lives. Every moment is an opportunity to wake up and stop sleepwalking through our lives. Simply being alive to each moment as it presents itself rather than being transfixed by the contents of our heads is something we can all practice doing, as many times a day as there are moments. Becoming aware of our own mental weather and internal running commentary and habitual grumblings is a great stride forward in our spiritual development. We train in this practice of mindfulness, and start waking up to life as it is.

In _asana_ practice, we can become aware of our mental distractions, agitations and escapes. 'How long is the teacher going to keep us in this challenging pose? That noise outside is annoying. Why does my body not do what that person's body does? I must finish that report when I get home. What shall we have for dinner?' And then we catch ourselves, and we guide our attention, again and again, back to this body, this breath, this moment.

In meditation, we learn to observe passing thoughts as though they were people walking past a pavement café. We train in noticing them without becoming involved in a narrative, and we become familiar with our thought patterns – we realise that we are the one watching; we are not the thoughts.

Self-enquiry also means independent study such as exploring yoga texts and reading relevant books – taking the initiative to explore ideas, concepts and theories for ourselves. In this way we grow in independence, and learn to test the waters for ourselves.

<u>*Ishvara pranidhana*: Surrender to the Divine</u>

The final *niyama* is *Ishvara pranidhana* – surrender to the Divine. We can each choose what Divine means to us as individuals – it might mean 'God' to you if you're religious, but yoga is not a religion and not a dogma - so perhaps the most accessible way to perceive it is as a deep and abiding felt connection with Life itself; a sense that you are a part of the Universe, and the Universe is a part of you. We are all animated by the same force. (Throughout this book I will use the words Divine, Consciousness, Source, Being, Life, Presence and Universe interchangeably – they all refer to the same thing.)

'Surrender' can be a contentious word, especially if you've had to fight for what's right during your lifetime. It may be helpful to consider surrender as 'letting be'. Acceptance of what is, does not remove our ability to do our work in the world and try to make things better. In fact it facilitates it, because we can only start from where we are, so we might as well get honest about where that is!

So we can think of *Ishvara pranidhana* as finding a sense of connection and unity; acceptance of and engagement with each moment as it arises; and immersion into the Universe around us, knowing that we are it and it is us. This state of being – this surrender to the Divine – comes to us in glimpses, as a sense of utter peacefulness and connection, complete unity, as practice deepens and unfolds.

The *niyamas* – personal observances - are about our relationship with ourselves and our inner life. Living with the values of cleanliness and order (*saucha*), contentment (*santosha*), enquiring into our own inner state (*svadhyaya*), being enthusiastic and disciplined in our projects (*tapas*), and feeling a sense of connection with life itself (*Ishvara pranidhana*), makes for a far more pleasant and equanimous environment inside our own heads!

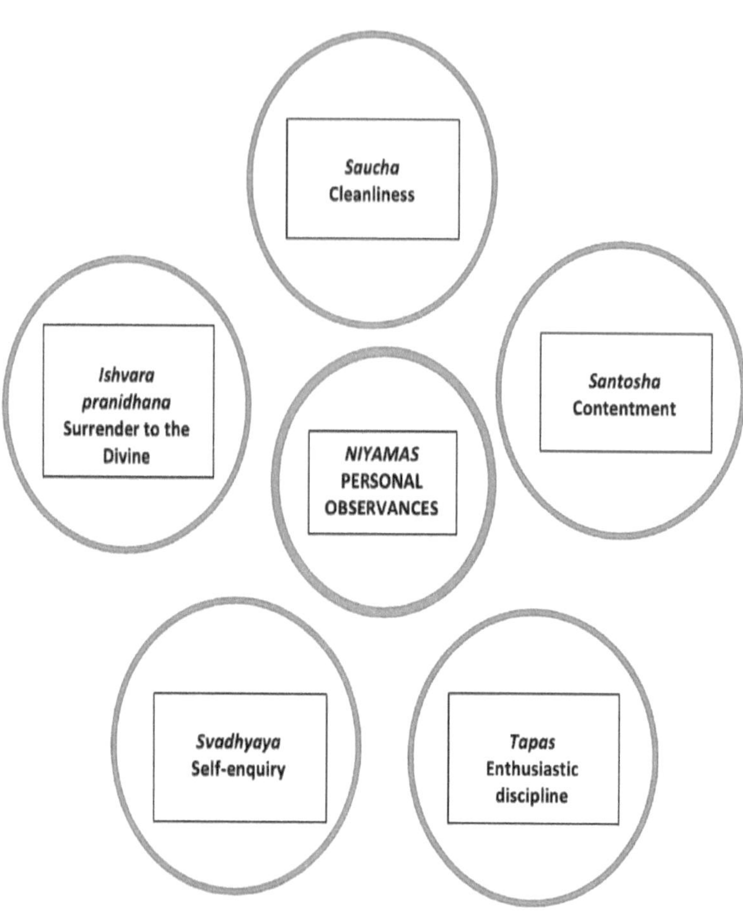

Saucha
Cleanliness
Santosha
Contentment
Ishvara pranidhana
Surrender to the Divine
NIYAMAS
PERSONAL
OBSERVANCES
Svadhyaya
Self-enquiry
Tapas
Enthusiastic discipline

The Eight Limbs of Yoga

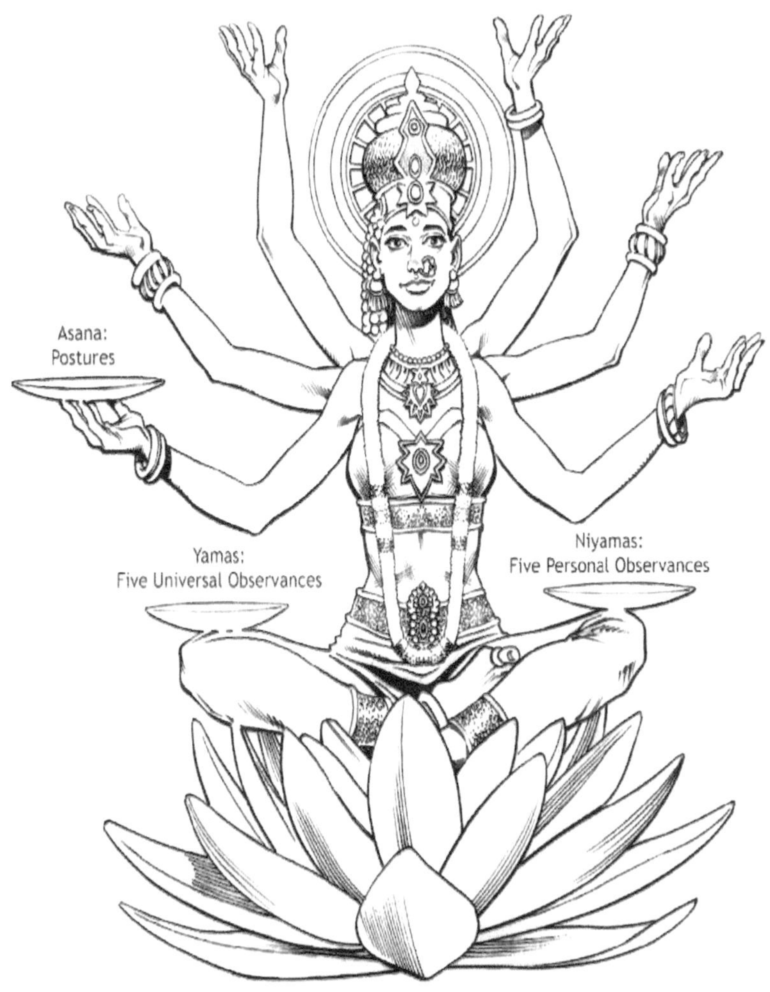

he limbs of yoga lead us progressively inwards. From the universal and

T personal values of the *yamas* and *niyamas*, we then move to taking care of our bodies with the third limb, *asana*.

The word *asana* – meaning seat – describes the physical postures of yoga.

The traditional reason for practising *asana* is to cultivate a strong, healthy, supple body, so that we can sit comfortably for longer periods in meditation and so access our inner sense of being. These bodies are our homes, and the practice of *asana* helps to keep them comfortable and well throughout our lives. It keeps our spines youthful and allows *prana*, the life-force, to flow and circulate freely in our bodies. It doesn't matter one iota if a body is stiff, or out of shape, or inflexible. It doesn't matter what a body looks like, or how old it is. We start where we are; the practice will meet us there.

As we will explore further in the next chapter, our mind-body connection is a two-way street. It is the case that our minds tell our bodies (both consciously and subconsciously) what to do - when we are stressed our brains will inform our bodies that they should be in a state of alert, ready to fight or flee, and so our muscles contract accordingly. Yet it is also the case that our bodies can inform our state of mind. If we find ourselves in a state of stress, with the tight muscles, raised shoulders, and frowning face which that induces, we have the ability to override the entire system simply by becoming aware of areas of tension in our bodies and consciously relaxing those muscles. If we do this, our brains recognise the relaxed body language and get the message that actually, there's no cause for alarm. The fight or flight response steps down, and we return to feeling more relaxed.

If you **mimic** a relaxed and happy state with your body, face and breathing, your brain and nervous system have no choice but to follow suit. *Asana* teaches us to be in a more relaxed state as our default setting.

When we're new to yoga we may perceive ourselves as only our bodies. In time, as subtle awareness develops through practice, we become attuned to a quieter part of ourselves and might start to feel that although we HAVE a body, we are much more besides.

A yoga practice draws us gradually further inwards to a still point within. However, for most of us when we're starting out it's enough of a challenge to simply keep our heads where our bodies are, and this is what asana trains us to do. By beginning with the movements of the body, combining them with breath, we develop concentration and quieten our minds. Gradually this physical practice becomes a moving meditation, inviting us inwards to explore the more mysterious parts of ourselves. This is what sets *asana* apart from gymnastics, Pilates and other forms of body-conditioning. The Yoga Sutras advise us that a yoga *asana* must have the qualities of *sthira* (steadiness) and *sukha* (ease); that is, we should be able to maintain the posture without forcing or straining. Our breath is our guide at all times – we must be able to breathe *dirgha (long)* and *sukshma* (smooth) in the physical shape. If breathing becomes restricted or laboured, then we are efforting too hard and should revert to a modified or less intense version of the posture. Movements within an *asana* practice should follow the breath – it is not enough to simply combine breath and movement as they can quickly become mechanical. The breath leads, and the movement follows. For example, in a simple practice of raising and lowering arms, the sequence would be as follows:

1 – Begin inhaling
2 – Begin raising arms
3 – Finish raising arms
4 – Finish inhaling
5 – Begin exhaling
6 – Begin lowering arms
7 – Finish lowering arms
8 – Finish exhaling

It's as though the breath is the envelope, and the movement is the contents. This method was advocated by the great teacher Krishnamacharya (1888 – 1989) the father of modern yoga. It means that we must concentrate intensely during practice, so helping our minds to become quiet and undistracted.

With this accomplished, then we may learn to shape our breath in the *asana*, perhaps emphasising or extending a particular phase of the breath (see chapter 6). Eventually we may add *bandhas* (see chapter 11).

An advanced yoga practice is nothing to do with what kind of complex *asana* you can get your limbs into, but how focused you can remain on your breath, the sensations, the flow of subtle energy within you, and the present moment. Someone who is standing on their head with their legs in lotus, but with their breathing all over the place and their mind on what they're having for dinner, is not really practising yoga at all. Someone who is chair-bound but is breathing long and smooth – *dirgha sukshma* (see chapter 6) – with their mind utterly absorbed in their practice as they bend forwards just a few degrees, can truly be said to be practising advanced *asana*. Yoga in the true sense is not about achieving some physical goal - it's a lifelong psycho-spiritual journey.

<u>Yoga and the spine</u>

The spine is an extraordinary structure which both provides support for the frame of the entire body, and also houses a safe channel through which the spinal cord passes, from the brain all the way to the lower back. This strong, flexible column comprises 33 individual bones or vertebrae in five regions.

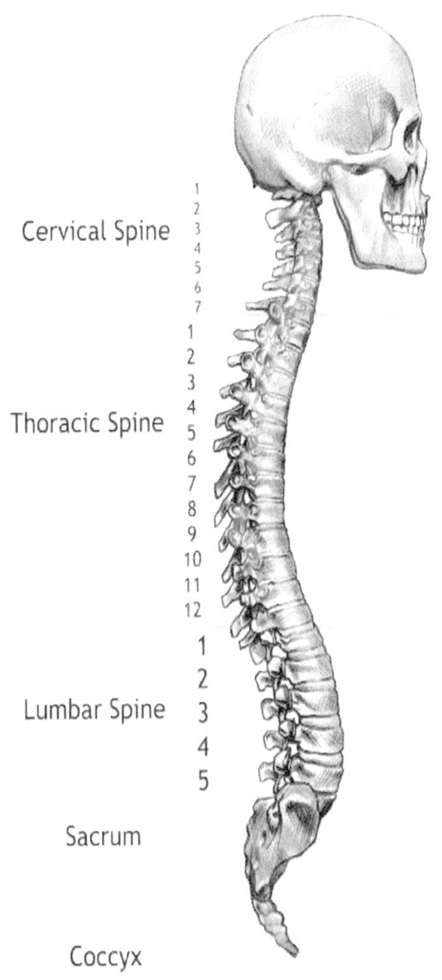

1 - Cervical spine C1-7

The skull rests atop the Atlas bone, which in turn is supported by the Axis bone. The Axis has a spigot-like bony projection which forms a pivot joint with the Atlas, allowing for mobility of the skull. Five further cervical vertebrae form the neck. The seventh cervical vertebra can be felt as a bony bump at the base of the neck if you lower your head forwards. This is the most mobile and also the most delicate part of the spine – the cervical vertebrae are a fraction of the size of the lumbar vertebrae as they are only required to carry the weight of the head (around 6kg). The natural curve that they form is lordotic, meaning that there is a convex hollow at the back of the neck.

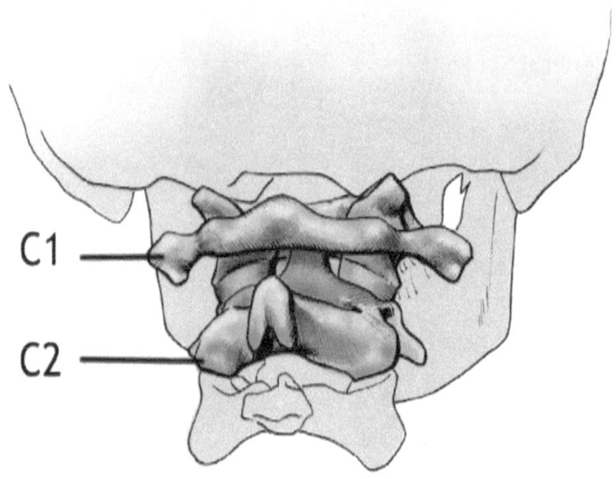

2 – Thoracic spine T1-12

The twelve thoracic vertebrae comprise the region from the base of the neck to the waist, and this is where the ribs are attached. They are larger than the cervical vertebrae and the greatest range of motion here is in twisting and side-bending movements. The natural curve formed here is kyphotic, forming an arc which rounds outwards to the back of the body.

3 – Lumbar spine L1-5

The five large lumbar vertebrae in the lower back primarily allow for greater weight support, and forward and back bending movements. Their natural curve is lordotic.

4 – Sacrum S1-5

The triangular bone at the base of the spine, roughly the size of the palm of your hand, is actually comprised of five fused bones. This is where the spine connects with the two iliac bones - the wings of the pelvis - to create the whole pelvic girdle. When we bend forwards or backwards, the sacrum 'nods' slightly (just a few millimetres) in relation to the iliac bones to facilitate that movement.

5 – Coccyx C1-4

Like the sacrum, the bones of the coccyx or tailbone are fused. Most people have four sections, but some have three and some have five. Unlike the rest of the spine, these bones do not have a hole through which spinal nerves pass. A 'leftover' from our ape ancestors, it serves no purpose and its absence generally creates no issues in the rare event that it has to be removed due to disease.

Between each pair of vertebrae there is a tough, spongy disc filled with a gel-like substance, which act as shock absorbers.

The vertebrae fit together in a series of chain-like links called facet joints, and these determine the range of motion in each area of the spine.

The spiky projection at the rear of each vertebra (which you can see and feel with your fingers when you bend forwards) is called a spinous process. This is where muscles attach, and they act as protective armour for the delicate spinal cord which runs through the cavity between the body of the vertebrae and the spinous processes. They also determine how different regions of the spine are able to move.

The curves of the spine and articulation allowed by the individual vertebrae (rather than a straight, solid bone) make it very strong, mobile and resilient.

A well designed *asana* practice moves the spine in all four directions – forward, back, side to side, and twisting – and thus keeps it supple and mobile.

The spinal column houses not only the vital spinal cord, which is the superhighway of all the body's nervous system, but also the main channel of *prana* in the subtle body, the *sushumna nadi*, and the *chakras*, all of which we'll explore in chapter 12. For *prana* to flow freely and for us to live with optimum health, it's vital that the spine is kept mobile and nourished through appropriate movement. It has been said that 'you're as young as your spine', and it's impossible to understate the importance of looking after this astonishingly clever part of our bodies.

A well-designed *asana* practice appropriate to the individual also mobilises and lubricates the joints, promotes healthy muscles by improving their strength, flexibility, elasticity and responsiveness, and keeps the fascia of the body (which is the connective tissue covering our muscles, bones, organs and blood vessels) free and supple.

<u>The purpose of different types of *asana*</u>

Different categories of *asana* can bring about different effects within the body, energy, mind and spirit. Although there is a vast range of postures within each category, from the simple to the complex, and from the totally passive to the extremely physically demanding, we can broadly say the following.

Forward extensions (also known as forward bends) stretch the muscles of the back of the body and are calming to the nervous system.

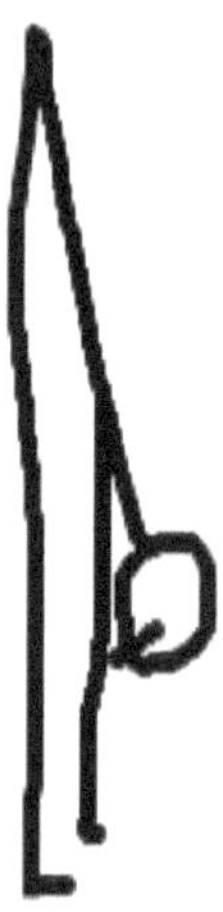

Back extensions (also known as backbends) stretch the front of the body and are invigorating.

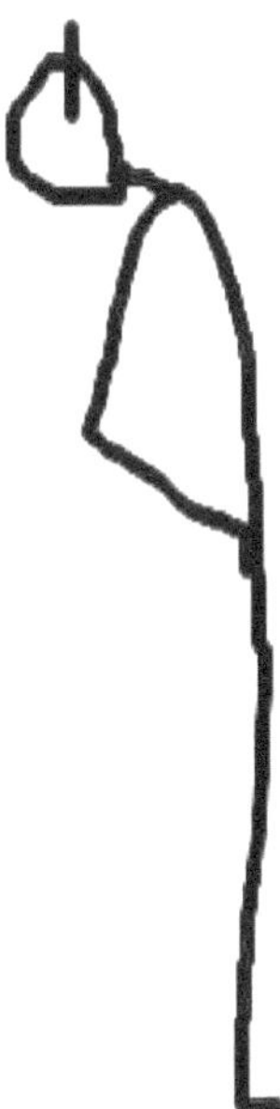

Side extensions release the often neglected muscles of the sides of the torso and ribcage and can help us to breathe more fully.

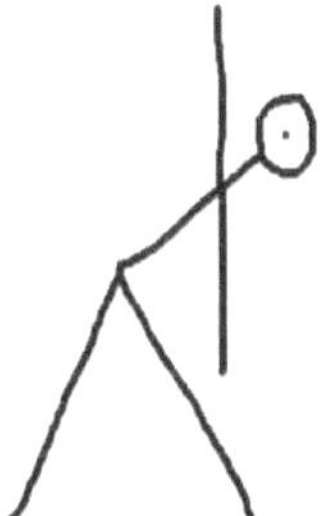

Twists gently massage and stimulate the internal organs.

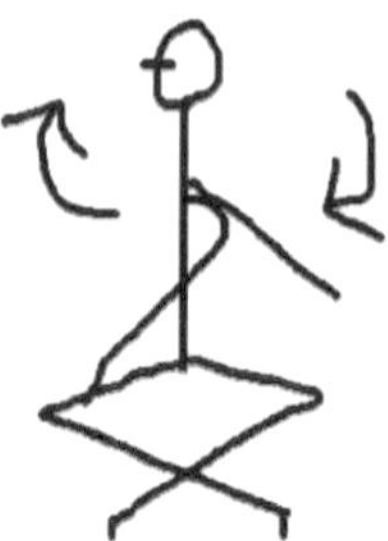

Inversions are stimulating in the short term (if active such as headstand) and calming in the medium to long term. They reverse the effects of gravity on the skeleton and organs, and assist the function of the lymphatic system.

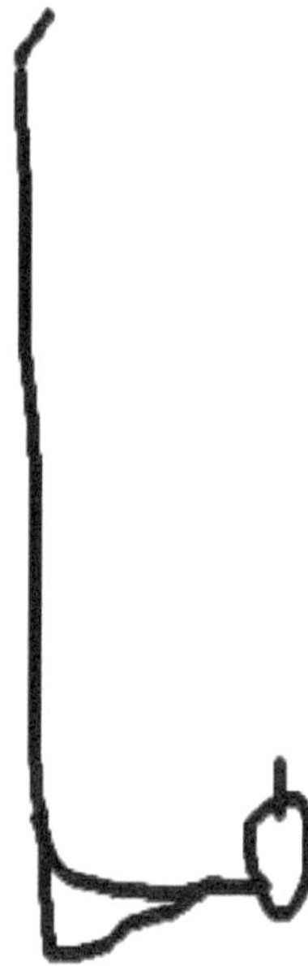

Leg balances improve concentration, strengthen the legs and hips, improve balance, and teach perseverance.

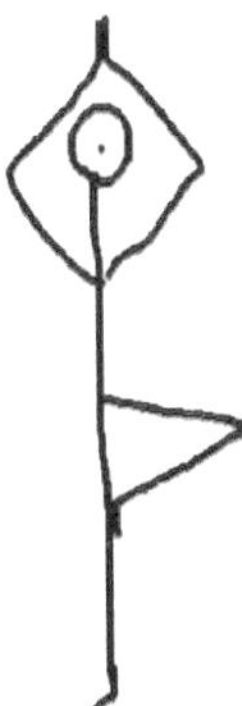

Arm balances improve upper body strength, teach perseverance and introduce a sense of playfulness.

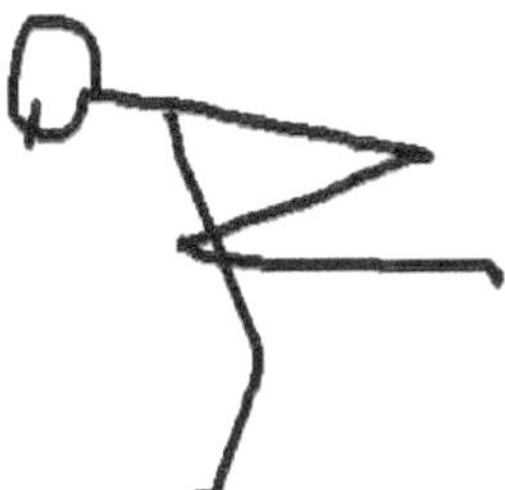

Restorative postures fully support the outer musculature of the body with props such as bolsters, folded blankets, firm foam blocks, belts, and chairs, so allowing the deep layers of postural muscles to completely release and relax.

All postures when practised regularly as part of a balanced and appropriate program in conjunction with the breath, can improve physical strength, mobility, comfort and suppleness, as well as confidence, concentration, proprioception, (awareness of where one's body parts are in space), mental calm, and sense of wellbeing. Appropriate movements of the spine keep the intervertebral discs nourished and healthy and facilitate the free flow of prana and optimal functioning of the spinal cord and nervous system.

A regular, intelligently targeted practice can also offer the following:

Greater bone density

Reduced blood presssure
Better sleep
Improved digestion/elimination
Reversal of functional illness ie Fibromyalgia and immune disorders
Reduction of symptoms of arthritis
Reduction or elimination of anxiety and depression
More energy
Reduction in scoliosis
Impetus to improve other lifestyle factors such as diet
Acceptance of oneself
Sense of self-worth
Greater connection with others
More positive outlook and appreciation for life
Greater longevity
Improved brain function
Ability to respond rather than react
Greater self-awareness
Reduced suffering in terminal illness
Greater self-trust
Connection with own intuition
Sense of peace

Whether you choose a dynamic form of *asana* practice or a slower paced style (and it can be extremely beneficial to vary your approach), even a few minutes of daily *asana* brings great benefits to how you experience your body, mind and energy.

The Eight Limbs of Yoga

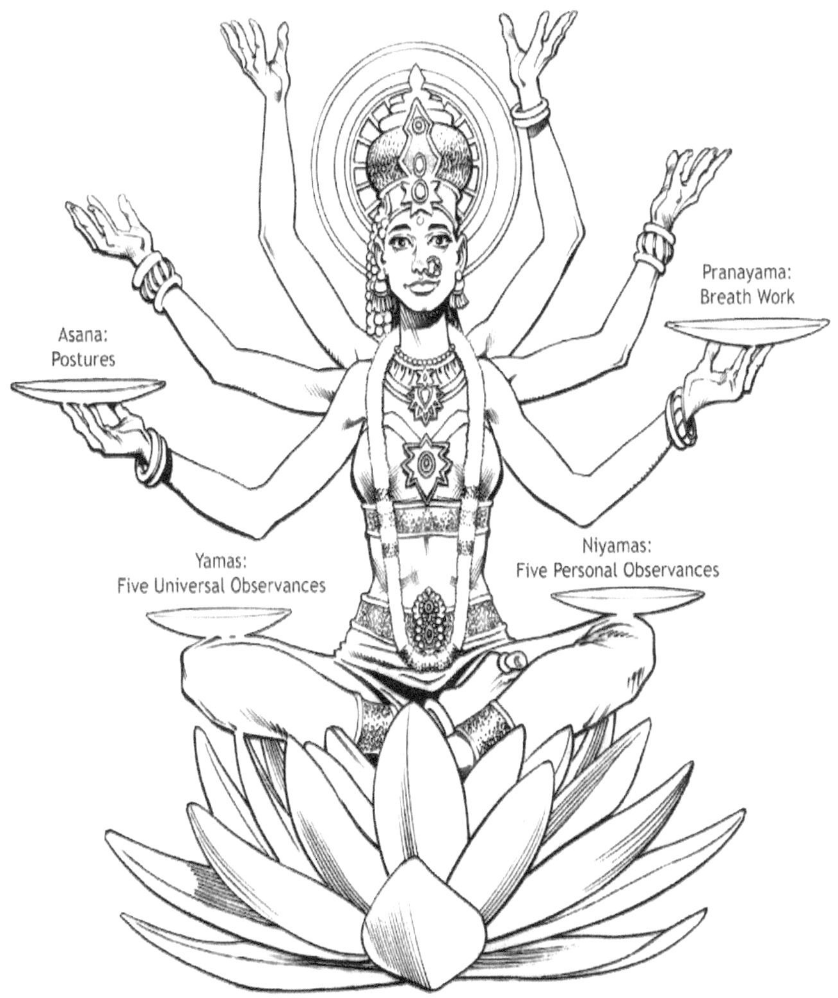

Moving towards the subtler aspects of yoga, the next limb we meet is *pranayama*.

Although we usually translate *pranayama* as 'breathwork', the literal meaning is extension (*yama*) of the life-force (*prana*).

When we practise full, smooth breathing, we balance the nervous system and bring it into a state of relaxed alertness – we are alive to the present moment, yet free from stress or tension.

How can something so simple as breathing do this?

Our breath is inextricably connected to our central nervous system. Within it there is a branch called the autonomic nervous system, which governs the body's automatic physiological processes so that we (thankfully) don't have to think about them. These are all the things that go on inside us: digestion, cell reproduction, heartbeat, immune responses and so on. Our breath is a unique function, in that it is both involuntary - we breathe without thinking about it - and also under our voluntary control. We can consciously alter the pattern of our breathing.

Our autonomic nervous system has two branches called the parasympathetic or 'relaxation response', and the sympathetic or 'readiness response'. Each time we exhale, the relaxation response is engaged; each time we inhale, the readiness response is engaged. When we are breathing fully and evenly and so are in a state of relaxed alertness, these two responses are equally matched, and for each invigorating inhale, there is an equal and opposite relaxing exhale. Both of these functions are vital, and when they are in balance – homeostasis – we feel good. When the nervous system is balanced, we naturally breathe fully and slowly, with a soft abdomen.

Now, think about what happens to your body when you feel stressed or anxious. What happens to your heart rate, your breathing, your muscles?

Stress and anxiety are the result of a perceived threat (note the word 'perceived' – our brains don't differentiate, and an imagined threat that we've worried our way into brings about exactly the same physiological changes as a physical risk to our lives does). The hypothalamus of the brain sends a message to the pituitary gland to say that there is danger. The pituitary gland signals to the adrenal glands to release the hormones adrenalin and cortisol, which pump into the bloodstream triggering a series of responses which prepare you to fight or flee: heart rate increases and blood is diverted away from some of the internal organs (like the digestive system) to your muscles so that they're primed for action; you might feel an urgent need to use the bathroom (to remove excess baggage in case of the need to to run); and your breathing becomes rapid, shallow and high in the chest.

What has happened? The brain perceived a threat, and told the nervous system to enter fight or flight mode – you are in full sympathetic activation, and that has automatically made your breath rapid and shallow.

In the case of acute stress – that is, dealing with an immediate emergency which requires action right now – that's exactly what needs to happen. Our bodies get primed to fight or flee, and we get out of the way of the oncoming car (or whatever threat has arisen) and save ourselves. Then, having taken fast an appropriate action, the relaxation response kicks in and we return to a normal, balanced state. All of these primal physiological changes happen in a split second – they have to, they're potential life-savers, so they happen BEFORE the assessing and reasoning parts of the brain come to the party.

Human life has changed dramatically in the last 500 years or so, but evolution takes a lot longer than that to catch up. Our brains aren't much different from 200,000 years ago, and for most of that time we lived in an immediate resolution environment, where if we were worried about a situation - about to get eaten by a predator, finding food, finding shelter - the anxiety created by that concern would go away as soon as it was resolved and we could return to a relaxed state. Our worry was a lifesaver. Since we became domesticated and industrialised however, we've given ourselves a bunch of new, different things to be concerned with, many of which can't be resolved immediately or even close to immediately. But we still have that same brain, which has not yet evolved to cope with such delays in worry resolution. Even more unhelpfully, our brains don't distinguish between real, in-your-face terror, and mind-created drama that will probably never happen. The physical results - that all too familiar feeling of stress and anxiety - are the same either way.

In modern life, stressors come thick and fast, and whilst our brains and bodies still perceive these alerts as real threats, we rarely need to respond with strong physical action. When the stress response is appropriate we run or fight, then the body returns to normal. But when the stressor is a traffic jam, or on a computer screen, or a mental state arising out of a personal situation, then what happens? There's nothing to flee, nothing to battle, and we become trapped in a prolonged state of fight or flight, and that's very bad news for our bodies. It increases our risk of heart disease, stroke, and digestive conditions such as ulcers, and causes weight gain. It messes up our sleep patterns, and can cause depression and anxiety disorders.

So at that point, we need to switch into the other side of the nervous system: the Parasympathetic Nervous System or the Rest and Relax response. When this is engaged our blood pressure and heart rate drops, our breathing is full and steady, digestion improves and we feel calm, at ease and relaxed.

But chronic stress – where we remain in an elevated stress state for long periods of time – is a disaster for our bodies. When we're getting out of the way of a speeding car, it's all about directing resources to the immediate situation. Longer term functions such as digestion, cell reproduction, and immunity are dialled way down. As the fight-or-flight state is only intended to be a short term thing, that's not a problem. But if we're constantly in that state, our other systems are suppressed for long periods, and that does becomes a huge problem.

Chronically elevated stress levels flood the body with the hormones adrenaline and cortisol. This internal environment creates raised blood pressure and inflammation in the body, and these conditions contribute heavily to life-threatening illnesses such as heart disease and many others.

Stress is just part of life. We can avoid some stressors, but a lot of them are simply part of the deal.

However, breathing is the golden ticket. You see, the conversation between the breath and the nervous system has a magic component: it's a two way street.

Yes, the autonomic nervous system tells the breath what to do. But the nervous system also responds to the breath, and will take its cue from the way in which we are breathing. And we can choose to take control of our breathing, which means that we can take control of our nervous system.

If we consciously choose to mimic relaxed breathing – slow and full – the nervous system gets the message that everything is ok, and it can step down from the state of high alert.

And THIS is why *pranayama* is such a vital component of yoga. Each time we consciously manipulate our breathing, we have the ability to profoundly affect our nervous system – and the nervous system affects EVERYTHING.

The literal translation of *pranayama* is 'extending the life force'. Given what we know about how devastating the effects of excess and chronic stress can be, this is no exaggeration. Those ancient yogis were onto something!

But I'm breathing all the time and I'm still alive – why do I need to change anything?

Clearly, we don't need to be taught how to breathe in order to stay alive – from the moment we take our first inhale as we're born, we know how to breathe without thinking about it. We breathe when we're busy doing other things, when we're asleep, and we can't actually STOP breathing voluntarily for any length of time.

But just because something is functioning, doesn't mean it's functioning optimally. As we grow up we come into contact with life's inevitable stressors, from losing sight of your parent in a supermarket, to playground squabbles, to exam nerves, to job interviews, to travelling to new places alone, to relationship breakdowns, to deaths of loved ones.... the list of the stressful events we encounter on life's journey is endless, and many of them are unavoidable. As we grow, we discover new ways of coping, we learn from our mistakes, and we collect all sorts of baggage which gets reflected in all aspects of our being. As we saw in chapter 1, we are multi-layered beings, and all the layers are interconnected.

Let's do an experiment. Stand up, and using only your body language, mimic a person who is sad and depressed.

Stay there in that body position, and notice what has happened to your chest, shoulders, abdomen and breathing.

Now, mimic a person who is happy, confident and full of life.

Stay there and notice what has happened to your chest, shoulders, abdomen and breathing.

Which one felt better?

Can you see how your mood might affect your posture, and therefore your breathing?

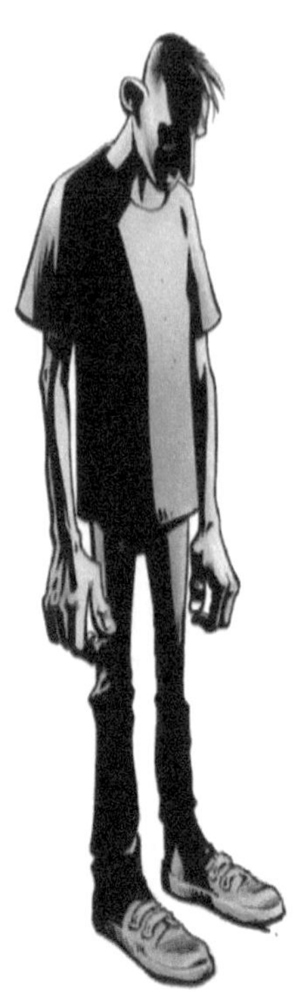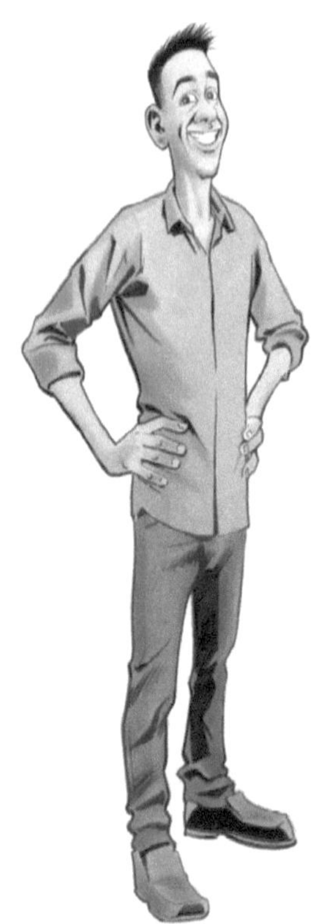

And knowing what we know about the two-way conversation between the breathing and the nervous system, can you see how your posture and your breathing might affect your mood?

So breathing well makes us feel better, but is that it?

The conversation between the breath and nervous system is not the only two-way street in the human body. Our minds and bodies are inextricably linked, and modern science is now catching up with what practitioners of yoga have known experientially for a long time: the mind-body connection is phenomenally powerful, and our quality of mind has a profound effect on the wellbeing of our bodies and ability to heal.

Personally I wouldn't want to live in a world without modern medicine. I could not be more grateful for it, when it is needed, and it is simply brilliant in acute illness and injury. But it often draws a blank when it comes to chronic illness brought about by lifestyles which have evolved at a pace which massively outstrips biological evolution. We are cave people living space age lives, and the stressors of modern living require a holistic approach to bring us back into balance.

So if you can manage and reduce stress, and thereby positively impact your health, with something as simple and accessible and free as learning to breathe more effectively – why on Earth wouldn't you?

<u>The Mechanics of Breathing</u>

When we breathe, fresh air containing oxygen enters the lungs, and stale air containing the waste gas carbon dioxide is removed.

Our two lungs are slightly different in size – the right lung is larger, comprised of three lobes, and accounts for 55-60% of lung capacity. The left lung is smaller and has only two lobes, to allow space for the heart. Beneath the lungs sits the diaphragm, which is a smooth, dome-shaped muscle attached to the ribs, sternum and spine. It is attached to the lungs by a double pleural membrane, which has a thin layer of pleural liquid sandwiched between the layers. This liquid creates a surface tension that keeps the membranes stuck together, in a similar way to water between two panes of glass.

When we inhale, the diaphragm muscle contracts and flattens out, which results in it moving down and pulling the bottom of the lungs down with it. (The external intercostals, pectoralis minor, sternocleidomastoid and scalenes also contract to move the ribs up and out.) This increases the volume of space within the lungs, and therefore decreases the air pressure. To equalise this pressure, air rushes in from outside (via the nostrils), and the result is that the lungs fill with air – an inhale. Although the lungs are contained within the ribcage, the lower abdomen normally expands as we inhale, due to the pressure of the descending diaphragm displacing the abdominal contents (also known as full diaphragmatic breathing or belly breathing).

When we exhale, the reverse occurs. The diaphragm relaxes and recoils upwards to its domed shape, the other aforementioned muscles also relax and release the ribs downwards and inwards, the abdominal muscles contract slightly, and the stale air passively moves out of the lungs, before the whole process begins again.

Diaphragm Action

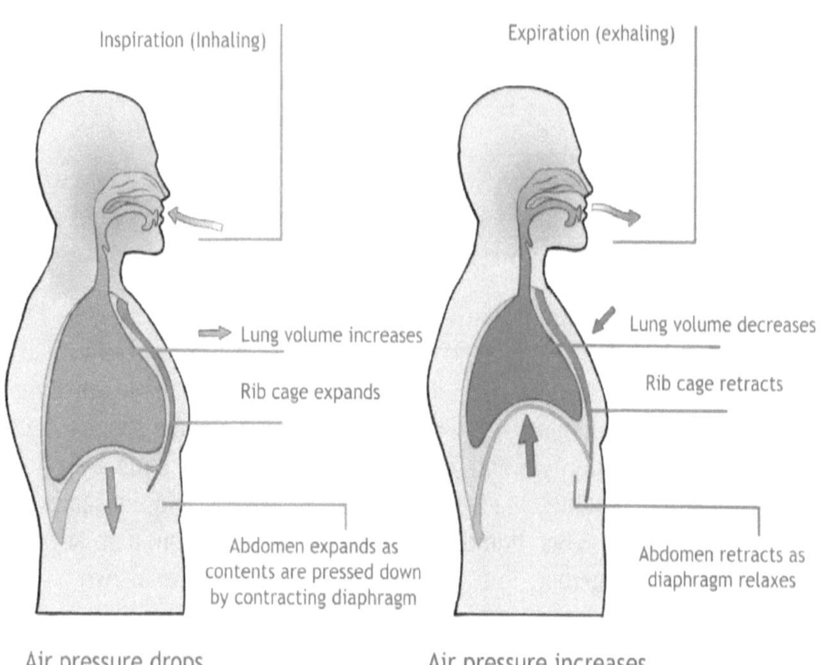

Breath Awareness and Development

Many of us aren't particularly aware of how we breathe until we begin practising yoga, and so simply cultivating breath awareness and developing a fuller breathing pattern is ample *pranayama* for a beginner. Even after decades of practice, this simple awareness of our breathing can be brought to our conscious attention numerous times throughout the day and at the beginning of every meditation and yoga practice.

Let's try it right now: without changing anything, simply pay attention to what your breath is doing. Where in your body are you most conscious of its movement? What qualities does the flow of your breath have: is it deep or shallow? Short or long? Smooth or jerky? Are the inhales and exhales the same length, or is one phase shorter than the other? Is there a slight pause at the top of each inhale and the bottom of each exhale?

You might find after a minute or so that this simple act of paying attention helps your breath spontaneously become slower, deeper, and more relaxed and even. What effect do you think that has on your nervous system?

Now see if you can allow the breath to expand all areas of your trunk in all three dimensions. As you inhale, allow your belly to soften and grow; the pelvic floor to subtly move down; the lower ribs to inflate to the front, back and sides like an umbrella opening up; the chest at nipple height to rise and open towards your shoulders; your collarbones to slightly lift. Can you even feel your back expand, and your spine grow a little taller?

As you exhale, all of these movements change direction, like your own internal tide. All of that expansion from the inhale now reverses and draws back to the centre point, and the pelvic floor lifts slightly, as the used air is gently pressed out of the body like a balloon emptying.Now see if you can bring your inhales and exhales to equal length by counting in your head.

What effect do you imagine all of that full and balanced breathing has on your nervous system?

This type of breathing is called *sama vrtti*, meaning 'equal fluctuation', and simply describes breathing evenly, with inhales (*puraka*) and exhales (*rechaka*) of equal length. It's vital to become established in maintaining *sama vrtti* breathing, before proceeding to work with extending phases of the breath and cultivating pauses (*kumbhaka* or retention), and then moving on to more advanced *pranayama* techniques. If *sama vrtti* was the only breathing technique you ever mastered, it would be enough.

<u>Cultivating the exhale</u>

When working with extending phases of the breath, beginning with the exhale is a wise approach which will optimise relaxation. Remember that the exhale is linked to the relaxation response – and we want to cultivate a relaxed state. When we extend the exhale, or suspend the breath at the end of an exhale, we emphasise that parasympathetic relaxation response.

Developing the inhale

Having extended the exhale, we can begin to do the same with the inhale, which is linked to the readiness response of the nervous system. When we expand the inhale, we give our bodies the maximum opportunity to receive and absorb *prana* in the form of oxygen to nourish every single cell in the body. By working with the inhale after we have first worked with the exhale, we ensure that we are first in a state of relaxation, then we increase the activation. The readiness response, when over-activated, becomes the fight or flight response – obviously not something we want from our yoga practice – and by working in this order we create a state of balance.

Honouring the pause

At the end of each inhale and exhale, there is a slight natural pause before the cycle returns in the opposite direction. It's like that moment of weightlessness when you're on a swing, before the return journey. At first it is enough to simply notice and honour the pause; as your proficiency in breathwork grows, you may practise extending first the pause after the exhale (which has a calming effect) and then the pause after the inhale (which has an enlivening effect). Retaining the breath in this way is called *kumbhaka*.

What the Sutras Say

Sutra 1.34 *Pracchardana vidharanabhyam va pranasya*

This sutra explains that one method for developing
a favourably disposed, serene and benevolent state
of awareness is to maintain the contemplative
state felt at the time of soft and steady exhalation
and during passive retention after exhalation.

Diaphragmatic breathing

Diaphragmatic breathing, or belly breathing as it is sometimes called, is a simple and effective way to optimise the balancing effects of full, even breathing. Picture the whole of your torso as made up of four segments:

Lower abdomen
Side ribs and upper abdomen
Chest (pectoral muscle area)
Upper chest (collarbone region)

You might find it helpful to imagine that each segment has an inflatable rubber ring around it.

To breathe diaphragmatically, inhale 'into' each of these regions (bottom to top); then exhale in the same order (bottom to top). Naming them in your head, 'belly, ribs, chest, upper chest' keeps a steady rhythm. Try to spread the inhale evenly across all four regions rather than rushing at the start and then running out of space. Exhale the same way.

Chest-to-abdomen breathing

This is a style taught by the great teacher Krishnamacharya. It emphasises the gentle massage effect breathing on the spine as it grows taller on the inhale and contracts on the exhale.

Inhale chest to abdomen – exhale abdomen to chest.

Inhale in this order, top to bottom:

Upper chest (collarbone region)
Chest (pectoral muscle area)
Side ribs and upper abdomen
Lower abdomen

And exhale in this order, bottom to top:

Lower abdomen
Side ribs and upper abdomen
Chest (pectoral muscle area)
Upper chest (collarbone region)

Try both of these methods for a few minutes each and see what differences you notice.

<u>Breathing as a yogic practice</u>

Yoga is a practice aimed at alleviating suffering. Life presents us with painful circumstances at times, and we can feel powerless; yet much of our suffering originates either from our own mental state, or arises as a mental reaction to painful situations. Our futile tendencies to want things to be a certain way; to cling on to some experiences and reject others; to resist reality, create suffering (which is optional) on top of pain (which may be unavoidable). Pain is the first arrow which may come from elsewhere; but our lack of skill in handling it means that we often shoot the second arrow at ourselves.

According to the yoga tradition the root of our suffering is a lack of spiritual understanding - an ignorance of our true nature as Life itself (see chapter 14). This is a profound concept, but yoga is nothing if not practical - we are given tools to remove the veil of ignorance which clouds our experience and makes things so much worse than they need to be. One of the most valuable of these tools is the ever-ready oasis of our breath. Even in the very darkest of places and hardest of times, our constant companion of breath is always with us.

How can something so simple as breathing help us deal with the kind of turbulence which life throws at us? The key is in the *way* we breathe; the qualities of expansion and subtlety - *dirgha sukshma* - which we bring to breathing can shift our minds, nervous systems, reactions and perspective into a very different place. As a result, our ability to cope with life's challenges is transformed. A shift in the quality of our breathing can do all of this, helping us to more skilfully navigate even the most troubling circumstances and alleviate our own suffering.

What the Sutras Say

2.50 *Bahya abhyantara stambha vrittih desa kala samkhyabhih paridrstah* **dirgha suksmah**

2.52 *Tatah ksiyate prakasa avaranam*

'*Pranayama* has three movements: **prolonged and fine** inhalation, exhalation and retention; all regulated with precision according to duration and place.... (it) removes the veil covering the light of true knowledge and heralds the dawn of wisdom.'

dirgha - long, expansive

suksmah (pronounced sukshma) - subtle, soft, fine, smooth

Prana-yama: extending the life-force

As the breath awareness practice develops, we can start to explore more particular types of *pranayama*. Here are a few of the more common styles – I recommended that you learn these with the in-person guidance of a qualified and experienced teacher.

Ujjayi

Meaning 'victorious breath', *Ujjayi* is a style of breathing common in Astanga and Vinyasa yoga, as well as other Hatha yoga styles. By slightly constricting the glottis at the back of the throat, you naturally slow down the breath. The action creates a slight snoring or ocean-wave like sound, and this helps to give the mind a focus of attention. You also take in more air with a slower breath, increasing the energy flow needed for a more dynamic yoga practice.

Nadi Shodhana

Nadi Shodhana means 'nerve cleansing', and is also known as 'alternate nostril breathing'. Using the thumb and ring finger of the right hand, you open and close alternate nostrils. The left nostril is related to the relaxation side of the nervous system, the right nostril to invigoration (more about that in chapter 17). For this reason we generally begin and end the practice by exhaling through the left nostril, as this creates the most calming effect.

Sitali

Sitali is a cooling breath. The tongue is rolled into a tube shape and you inhale through the tunnel created, then close the mouth and exhale normally through the nose. By 'drinking' in the cooled air in this way, we can reduce overheating in the body – particularly useful during hot weather and menopause.

Brahmari

Also known as 'humming bee breath', *Brahmari* is great for calming the nervous system and creating hormonal balance by influencing the hypothalamus, pineal and pituitary glands. You begin by inhaling normally through your nostrils, and then humming on the exhale – like saying 'om' but with the mouth closed and the teeth parted so your jaw is relaxed. Once you have the hang of that, you place your thumbtips over the tragus (central cartilage flap) of the ears and rest the other fingers on your face. You then close your eyes and gently press your ears closed, so that now when you hum the exhale out, you feel the whole skull resonate. This has a profoundly calming effect, and done correctly is one of the most healing breath practices yoga has to offer.

The following *pranayama* practices are more vigorous - please ensure

that you learn them under the guidance of a qualified and experienced teacher.

Viloma

The term *viloma pranayama* has described a few different styles of practice in different traditions; however, the version you are most likely to encounter is also known as 'ladder breathing'. You begin by cultivating *sama vrtti Ujjayi* breath, of an equally balanced inhale and exhale with a slight constriction in the glottis. Then, working first with the exhale, you begin to pause a few times, as though you're letting the air out of a balloon a little at a time, pinching it shut in between. It feels a little like your breath is walking down steps. Once comfortable taking four or five momentary pauses during the exhale, you then repeat the process with the inhale, sipping the breath in through the nostrils a little at a time. The overall effect of this is that you dramatically slow down the time it takes to perform one full round of breath. Depending on how the practice is structured, you can create a calming, enlivening, or balancing effect with *viloma pranayama*.

Kapalbhati

Kapalbhati means 'skull-shining breath', and is technically one of the *shatkarma* purifying techniques (chapter 11). After taking a full inhale, you quickly pull the belly back to press the air out through the nostrils in a series of short, rapid exhales. There is a short inhale after each exhale, which happens passively and without force. *Kapalbhati* creates a clearing effect in the mind, as well as strengthening the abdominal muscles and massaging the lower abdominal organs, making it a useful tool if constipated.

Bhastrika

Similar to *kalpalbhati*, *bhastrika* emphasises both the the exhale and the inhale. Whereas the inhale arrives passively in *kapalbhati*, in *bhastrika* it is drawn in actively, earning it the name 'bellows breath'. This makes it very invigorating, and whilst it is said to be beneficial to the circulatory and immune systems, it may cause some light-headedness and has a number of contraidications including asthma and high blood pressure, so must be practised with caution.

Learning to breathe optimally brings about profound changes in our mental and emotional state, nervous system, lung efficiency and overall health. *Pranayama* gives us the tools to influence our entire state of being at any time, no matter where we are or what the circumstances, for free. Think about it – taking a breath is the first, and last, thing we ever do. Throughout our lives we never stop doing it, and if you think that concentrating on your breathing is boring, imagine being unable to breathe for just one minute and see how boring you'd find it then! But just because we do it automatically, doesn't mean we do it properly– in fact most of us don't breathe well at all – and we each have the capacity to improve our breathing and therefore our lives. Breath is life, and if you're hardly breathing, you're hardly living.

The Eight Limbs of Yoga

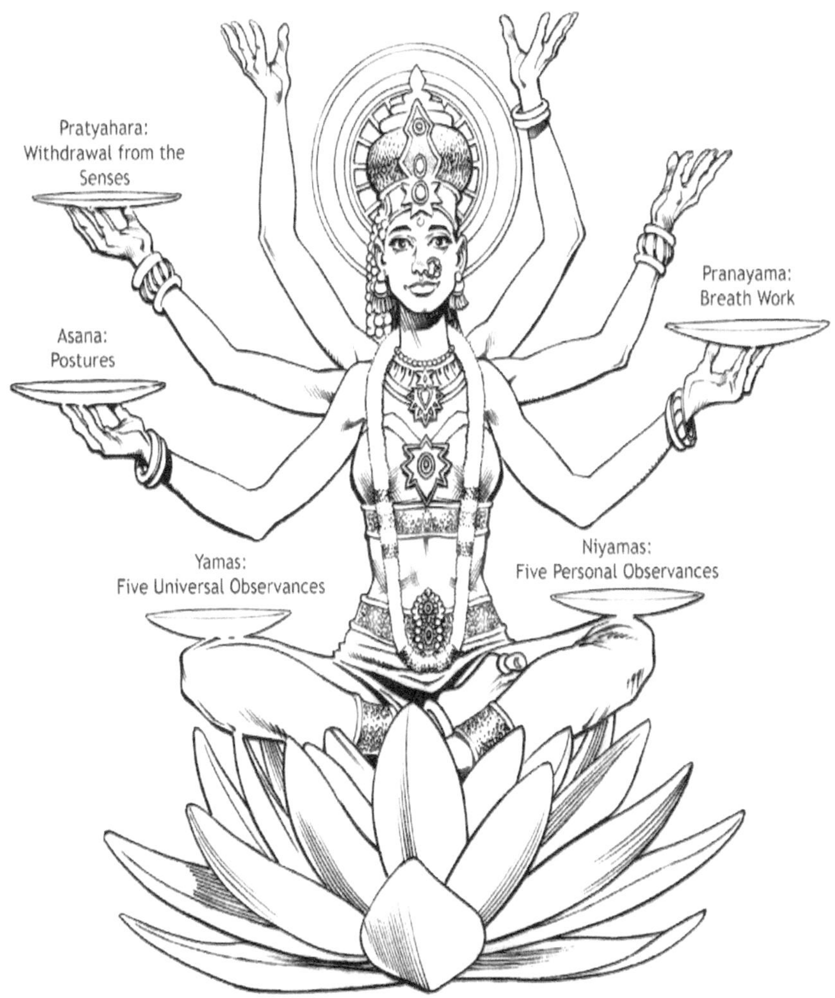

So far we have looked at the first four limbs of yoga.

You might have noticed by now that each of these limbs of yoga is gradually moving from the more tangible to the more inwardly focused; from the gross to the subtle (the word 'gross' in this instance meaning 'obvious', not 'disgusting'). With the fifth limb of *pratyahara*, we begin the journey within.

As we weave the *yamas* and *niyamas* into our lives, practise *asana*, and develop our *pranayama* breathing, we start to feel more centred and less scattered. In this way we begin to cultivate *pratyahara* or 'withdrawal from the senses'. It's a little like the ocean – it might be choppy and splashy on the surface, subject to the changing winds and passing traffic, but when you go deeper down it gets smoother and calmer. There's still movement, but it's less frenetic. As we move into a state of *pratyahara*, we are less easily distracted by external occurrences and irritations, and our focus of attention draws closer to our centre, much like a sheepdog herds their flock into a central location. *Pratyahara* is, in a gross sense, about ignoring distractions. However, being told to 'just ignore' something is about as helpful as the old example of being told not to think of a pink elephant – it's pretty hard to 'do' a negative. So we take our minds off sensory distractions by gathering our attention and focusing it on something in particular, such as movement and breathing – we become 'mindful' of what we're doing, and therefore less easily distracted by every passer by, sound, itch, smell, or thought of lunch. *Pratyahara* is therefore not so much something you 'do', as a state which arises as a result of other practices.

As the fifth limb, *pratyahara* is the bridge between the more outwardly focused limbs which we have met so far on our outer quest (*bahiranga sadhana* – outer limb practice), and the subtler last three which comprise the inner quest (*antaranga sadhana* – inner limb practice).

The word itself is comprised of *prati*, meaning 'to turn away from', and *ahara*, meaning 'that which we take in'; so in a state of *pratyahara*, we turn away from external influences. Our diet is not only what we eat, but everything that we take in via our senses. Some things that our senses deliver to us we have control over – what we choose to watch on TV, for example – whereas others are out of our control, such as the noise from passing cars. The modern age offers more distractions than humans have ever experienced. Social media and advertising have impaired our ability to focus for more than a few minutes, and unless we deliberately make the decision to disengage from external stimuli, there is always something vying for our attention.

We can begin to feel a sense of withdrawing attention from the non-helpful by exercising wise discrimination (*viveka*) over what we invite into our lives. Sometimes we may not be consciously aware that something – or someone – has a detrimental effect on us. By checking in with ourselves throughout the day and noticing when we feel uplifted and nourished, or flat and drained, we can do the detective work as to what contributes to our wellbeing, and what detracts from it. It might be that after watching the news headlines you feel informed, but then after continuing to watch a half hour of analysis and talking heads you feel depressed. You might notice that interacting with this person puts a spring in your step, but that person leaves you feeling pessimistic or dissatisfied. Perhaps you reduce the amount of time you spend scrolling social media and trim your feed to include only contibutions which are truly interesting or uplifting. These are the things we have agency over – we can withdraw our time and attention from the influences which harm us. We might then choose to use that newly freed-up time and attention more wisely, choosing to soothe and nourish our senses with more helpful influences and impressions, perhaps by sitting in nature without a phone in hand, or creating a more peaceful environment at home by tidying up and lighting some incense. We can also create helpful inner impressions by doing visualisation practices and reading inspiring books. These things start to create the internal conditions for a more spacious, calmer way of being.

True *pratyahara* develops over time as a by-product of practising the earlier limbs, particularly *asana* and *pranayama*, as well as the next limb, *dharana* (remember, the limbs are presented sequentially, but in practice they are interwoven). We can't pay attention to **everything**, and paying close attention to **anything** requires that we withdraw our attention from other things. By becoming intimately aware of our body's position and sensations in *asana* and consciously steadying our breathing so it becomes slow and rhythmic, our attention is withdrawn from other sensory distractions. We naturally begin to experience sense withdrawal by practising *sthiram sukham asanam* (steady ease in the posture). Cultivating *ujjayi* breath gives us an auditory focus for our hearing; resting our eyes at a certain *drishti* (gaze point) provides a visual focus, so that we are not distracted by external sounds and movements. Gradually we become so absorbed that our senses are no longer drawn to external objects. *Yoga nidra*, which we'll explore in chapter 11, is a deep (and very enjoyable) practice of *pratyahara*.

In time this state of inward focus starts to influence everyday life. We might find that we are less easily distracted at work, or less irritated by external factors which are out of our control. We might find an increase in our capacity to simply ignore mundane annoyances which we can do nothing about. We may develop greater willpower and become clearer in our thinking. The mind starts to feel less like an out of control puppy whose attention is temporarily caught by everything which passes it, and more like a mature and friendly well-trained dog, who barks only when necessary, and rests peacefully at other times, ignoring irrelevant distractions.

Pratyahara is the gateway between the yoga you can see from the outside, and the yoga which can't be observed by an onlooker. It is the gateway between the outer and inner self.

'If a man's reason succumbs to the pull of his senses, he is lost.'

BKS Iyengar

The Eight Limbs of Yoga

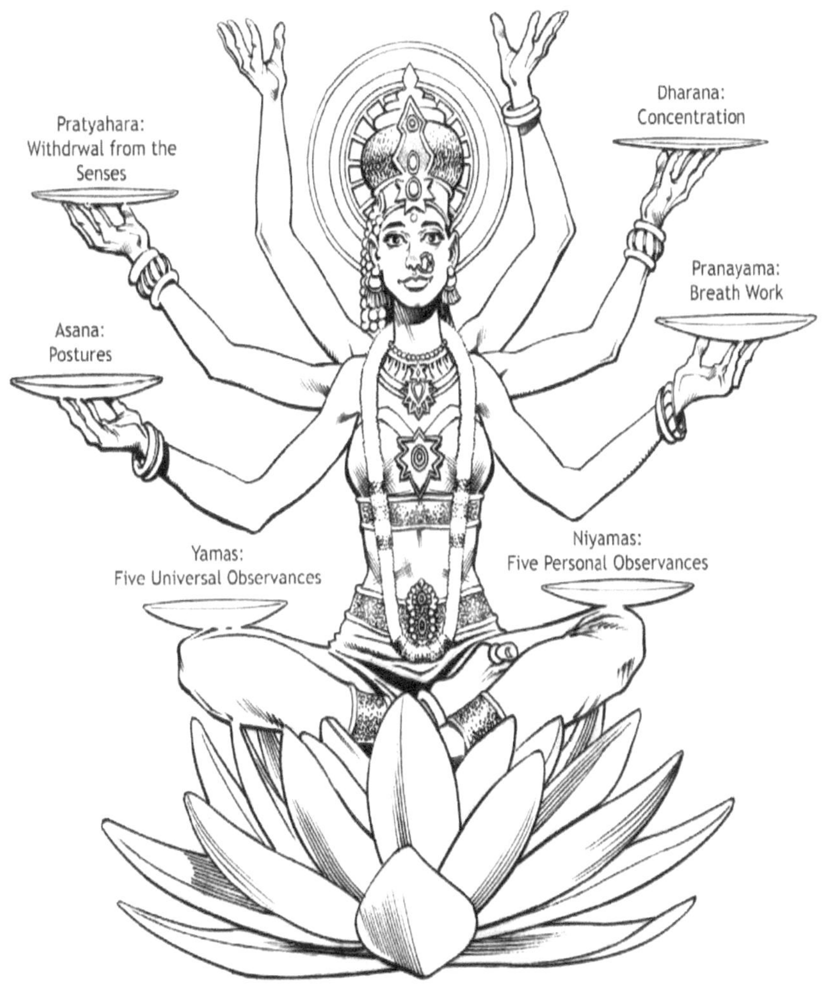

he sixth limb of yoga is *dharana* or focused concentration. In our modern world of near-constant distractions this can be challenging, but concentration is like a muscle, and the more we practise the stronger it gets. Yoga offers tools to develop concentration, such as *mudra*, *drishti* and *trataka*, which will be explained in chapter 12, as well as many visualisation practices found throughout Yogic, Tantrik and Upanishadic texts. The simplest of *asana*, combined with full attention on breathing, is the way which most of us begin to practise *dharana* within the yoga context.

Concentration is the laser focused awareness of mind. (It can be helpful to think of concentration less in terms of being told to 'concentrate!' by a teacher at school, and more like concentrated orange juice – you are gathering up all your attention and mental faculties and condensing them into one area.) In intense concentration, external surroundings seem to fade away, and the object of concentration is the only point of illumination. In this state, the human mind is incredibly powerful and extraordinary things can be accomplished. This is what is meant by being in a state of flow – the task at hand becomes enormously enjoyable as we are so absorbed in it that the work seems to flow through us – we feel as though we are simply a conduit for a greater power. Most of us do not use our minds in this way – we are easily distracted, and a task which would take an hour with total concentration can take all day. Developing the art of concentration is enormously useful in our everyday lives, and more than that, it open us up to the more profound gifts of yoga. If we can concentrate, there is no end to what we can achieve in life, and without the ability to concentrate we cannot hope to fine-tune the awareness into a state of meditation.

Dharana is the first of the three limbs which relate specifically to the meditative practices of inner yoga. Collectively these three limbs are known as *samyama* or integration. *Dharana* is the beginning of our inner quest, the quest of the soul (*antaratma sadhana* – inner self practice).

In practising *dharana*, we consciously direct the attention towards a particular object. This may be an external object, such as a *yantra*, flame, flower, or natural scene; a *mantra* repeated either out loud or internally; or the *chakras*, tip of the nose, or tip of the tongue. It can also be our own body in an *asana*. One very commonly used object of concentration, which is considered a sacred object, is our own breath – which is very useful, as we always have it with us. Most people need an object to concentrate on – it is very difficult to concentrate on nothing, and the average mind will simply dart manically around everything that it encounters.

Dharana practice reduces the interruptions of our minds, and brings them under control into a state of right attention. In the yoga tradition, our minds exist in any of five states:

Kshipta – scattered, messy, totally undisciplined, grasping randomly at external desires.

Mudha – tired, stuck, unmotivated, dull, or foolish, lacking in intelligence.

Vikshipta – attempting to concentrate but agitated, distracted.

Ekagrata – single-pointed awareness, keenly focused, right attention, concentrated, clear and accurate perception.

Nirodha – suspension of mental fluctuations. All aspects of mind are harnessed and in service to a greater purpose. (Remember that second *sutra - yogah citta vrtti nirodhah* – yoga stills the fluctuations of the mind.) In this meditative state of awareness we can be performing actions, but it's as though we are a conduit for pure Being – the work flows through us.

When the state of *ekagrata* is discovered for a sustained period of time, we are ready to enter the next limb of yoga.

The Eight Limbs of Yoga

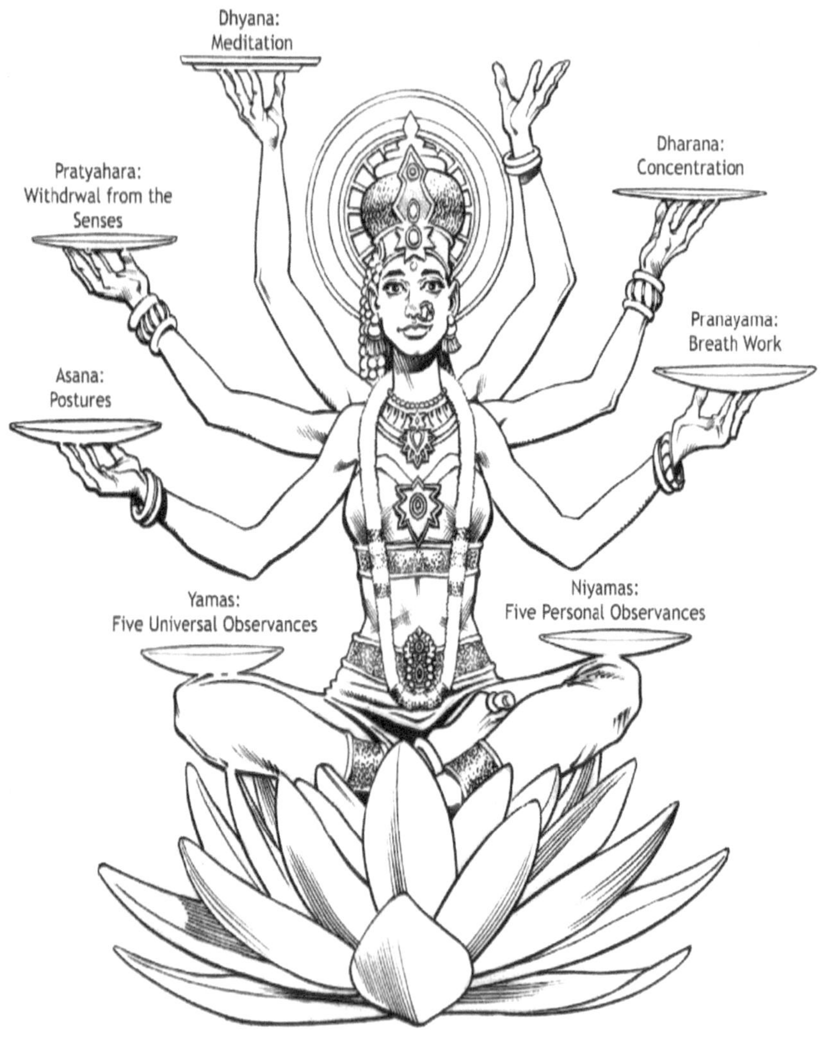

A s we come into the subtlest realms of yoga practice, we meet the seventh limb, meditation.

Meditation - *dhyana* - has received a lot of attention in the West in recent years, with excellent reason. Whether we're looking simply to find a little space in our busy minds and reduce anxiety, or enter into a state of blissful union with the Universe, meditation is the master key.

You can't actually 'do' meditation – it's a state of being which results from withdrawing our attention from external distractions and laser-focusing the mind. Sitting down without focusing on anything and and drifting off into a pleasant reverie is not meditation, it's daydreaming; so we first have to bring the activities of mind under control and learn to concentrate. The crossing over point between *dharana* (concentration) and *dhyana* (meditation) comes when we retain the point of awareness, but the concept of ourselves as separate from the object and the act of observation fall away, leaving only absolute awareness. So true meditation is not something we can wilfully 'do' – it's a state which arises as a result of practising over a long time period with enthusiastic dedication and regularity.

However, as we so commonly use the term 'meditation' to describe techniques, we'll continue with it here for the sake of practicality.

There are many different forms of meditation, and different schools of philosophy (ie Yoga, Tantra, Buddhism) all have their methods which may include taming the mind with *mantra*, visualisation, or focused gazing. The simplest method is to sit and just observe your breath. When starting out, find a style that resonates with you, and then stick with it. It's generally best not to 'shop around' too much once you find a method you like, as it takes time for a practice to become familiar and to develop a degree of proficiency. Guided meditations and apps have become very popular these days, and whilst they can definitely be a useful tool for familiarising yourself with the process, it's important not to let them become a crutch. The state of meditation is already within you, and so finding it is not dependent on an external prop.

Practical Benefits of Meditation

Chronic stress is the underlying cause of a vast number of illnesses and health conditions – it is a plague of the modern age. Through breathwork and meditation we have the power to bring our nervous systems back into balance, and therefore to reinstate the optimal function of all of our body's systems. The branch of medicine called psychoneuroimmunology (the study of the interaction between psychological processes and the nervous and immune systems) has consistently shown that by taking advantage of the two-way street that is the mind-body connection with breathwork and meditation, we can reduce chronic stress and its disastrous, often fatal, results. That alone is ample reason to get a regular meditation habit. The knock-on effects of basic meditation include:

- Improved mental health, including reduced incidence of anxiety and depression.
- Reduced blood pressure.
- Reduced risk of stroke.
- Reduced risk of heart disease as well as other serious illnesses.
- Improved digestion.
- Improved sleep.
- Increased ability to deal with and be resilient to life's stresses.
- Increased sense of wellbeing.

<u>Common Obstacles and Pitfalls</u>

Little and often is key - it's better to practise for five minutes every day than to try to sit for half an hour once a week. Half an hour is a long time for a beginner, so it's important to build up gradually. In this way you will develop a habit that is realistic and enjoyable to stick with, as well as cultivate the ability to sit comfortably for longer and longer periods of time.

There are some common problems that new meditators encounter, such as:

I can't get my mind to keep still.

Don't worry! Busy minds are perfectly normal – in fact they're a feature of being human. It's not possible to 'make' your mind be quiet through force of will, and the harder you try, the more your mind will resist. Instead, the trick is to repeatedly return your attention to whatever you are focusing on, be that your breath, a *mantra* or something else. Thoughts WILL arise, but the process of training is to notice them without entering into conversation with them. At first you'll keep finding that you've engaged with a thought and it's turned into thinking. That's normal. As soon as you become aware of what's happened, just drop the story and return to your focal point. Training your mind is a lot like training a puppy to sit and stay, without running off in all directions at the slightest distraction. Understand that this IS a training process, and no-one is good at anything the first few hundred times they do it! You wouldn't expect to be able to run a marathon without ever having been for a jog, and this is no different.

I get bored.

Your mind may feel agitated and want to escape. Now more than ever, we're used to being entertained almost constantly during waking hours – think back to the last time you were on public transport. How many people were looking at their phones? In the modern world, the moment we feel bored or remotely uncomfortable there's an instant escape – we never have to tolerate just BEING with ourselves. Being bored and sitting with mental discomfort is a really healthy state to cultivate, and once your mind gets used to the idea that you're not paying attention to it, its noisy chatter becomes more like sporadic distant mumbling. The boredom stage is an important one to go through, because its around here that it dawns on you that **you are not your mind.** It's impossible to overemphasise the importance of this realisation. If you are able to watch your mind, then you can't be your mind. So who are you? You are the one who watches – the *drasta*, or witness. **This is a profound step**.

My legs go numb / my back or neck hurts.

Finding a meditation posture that is comfortable for your body is critical to your practice. If you're in physical agony you won't be able to concentrate, and besides, it's not healthy to endure agony! Refer back to the diagram of the spine in chapter 5, and notice how the lumbar spine curves inwards towards the belly. You need to preserve that natural curve, because otherwise other parts of your body will be forced to compensate – typically your chest will slump and your head will jut forward or 'hang' on your neck muscles, which gets uncomfortable very quickly. To correct this, start at the bottom.

In order for the lumbar curve not to flatten, your pelvis needs to have a slight forward tilt; so place a firm cushion or folded blanket under the rear half of your buttocks. It doesn't matter whether you sit cross-legged or not – no magic powers will be visited upon you if you possess one of those rare bodies which can comfortably sit in full lotus pose! Sitting with your back against a wall and your legs outstretched is perfectly fine, as is sitting in a chair with both feet flat on the floor; but whichever posture you choose, you will almost certainly need that elevating cushion or blanket under your buttocks. Your knees should be below your hips (use as much propping as you need for this to be the case) and your limbs symmetrically arranged. Here's a quick way to tell if your posture is respecting your lumbar curve: put your fingers on your spine, just below waist height. Now, tilt your pelvis forward and back. As you do so, you'll feel a little trough appear and disappear beneath your fingers. The trough means that your lumbar curve is intact, so prop up the back of your pelvis as much as you need to, in order to keep that in place. With your hips and lower back stabilised, the rest will more easily take care of itself as the remaining spinal curves naturally stack, with your head resting easily and upright at the top. It can be useful to imagine a string from the back of your tongue up through the top of your head to find a neutral neck alignment; similarly, you can imagine you are lightly pressing the back of your head into someone's hand, then draw your chin down very slightly. Your hands can rest wherever they feel most comfortable, with elbows bent and arms relaxed.

You may still find yourself losing your alignment from time to time, which will probably come to your attention in the form of back or neck soreness, or slumping. Simply make the necessary adjustments slowly and with minimal fidgeting so as not to further disturb yourself.

If you find your legs going numb, the normal reaction is to move them, but the problem is often further upstream – your sciatic nerve may be slightly squeezed from you sitting on it. Try leaning forward from your hips to release the pressure, and you'll probably find that the feeling returns almost immediately.

I don't have time.

Yes, you do. Sorry to be bossy, but you do, it's just a question of priorities. If you have time to watch TV, or go on social media, or scroll the news, or hit the snooze button, you have time to meditate for five minutes. What DOES help, though, is linking your new habit to something you already do – maybe right before you brush your teeth for example. First thing in the morning is generally best, because your mind hasn't yet had external stimulation and disturbance, and you're literally making it your priority by putting it first. Plus then it's done and you can feel calm and smug all day.

My kids / animals won't leave me alone.

Being a new parent is one set of circumstances that may prevent you from being a first-thing in the morning meditator – there's nothing like having a crying baby or a small child bouncing on your head to throw the best laid intentions out of the window. If you're a single parent with sleep deprivation and no support, I salute you for even wanting to try to find time. Only you know what might work in your daily schedule, but keep it small and managaeable and commend yourself for any and all efforts, even if it's taking just ten slow breaths before bed. And take comfort in the fact that they do get older, and one day you will have time for yourself again.

Older kids can normally cope with the concept that they are not to disturb you for a brief period. As for animals, once they've been let out to relieve themselves you might be surprised how quickly they settle if you ignore any attention-seeking antics. Often they love the peaceful energy and will quietly curl up right beside you!

A regular, dedicated meditation practice is a jewel worth cultivating. It's not always easy or blissful, and sometimes it's downright uncomfortable and annoying. Sitting with yourself is hard, and the temptation to seek distraction, entertainment or escape can be extremely strong! But it is also the ultimate form of *svadhyaya* (self-study); a kind of laboratory where we get to observe our habitual reactions, mental escapes and the nature of our mind chatter and self-talk. When we begin to understand ourselves on this level, we unlock a far greater capacity for growth and personal development than is possible in our day-to-day state. With regular practice, we can discover within ourselves an ever-present source of peace and equanimity – an inner retreat which was always there but which we never even knew existed, much less how to access it. That sense of an unwavering centre of peace feels, to me at least, like simultaneously having absolute expansive freedom and finally coming home.

<u>Meditation as a Higher Practice</u>

As fabulous as even the most basic of breathing and concentration practices is for our physical and mental health, the likes of Patanjali and the Buddha obviously weren't using meditation to manage stress from too many emails or rush hour traffic! And as entire schools of philosophy which have survived several millenia arose through what they discovered and shared, there's probably a bit more to it than calming down your mental chatter and feeling relaxed.

In the earlier limbs of yoga, effort is required. *Dhyana* – meditation -begins when *dharana* – concentration - evolves and practice becomes effortless; there is simply an uninterrupted flow of total awareness. It's important to remember that this is our natural state – our naked consciousness, if you like, before we clothe it in misapprehensions, identifications, attachments, aversions and insecurities. Although sustained effort is required in the earlier limbs in order to dial down these afflictions, there is no striving in discovering a state of meditation – it is not something which can be attained because **it's already within us**. It's a case of systematically stripping back the layers, to reveal the truth of who we really are.

Becoming one with the ultimate truth of existence which is revealed as a result of profound absorption in a meditative state, free from inner disturbances of our minds, is both the purpose and the state of yoga.

The Eight Limbs of Yoga

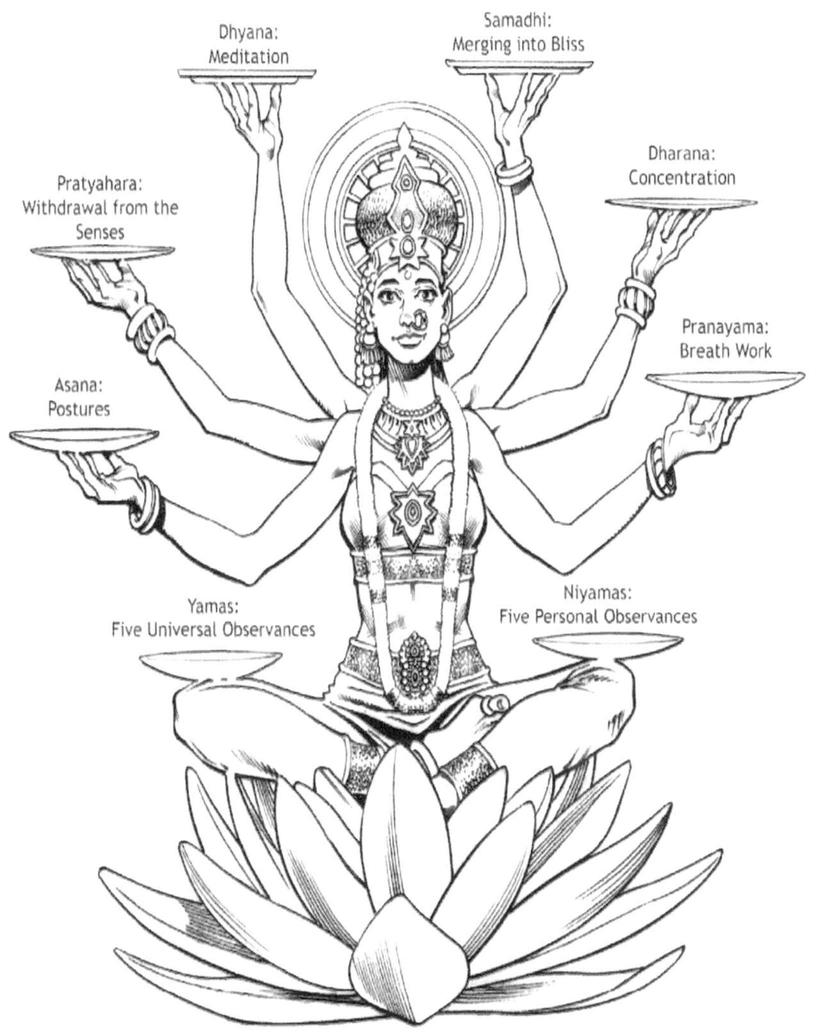

*S*amadhi is the eighth and final limb of yoga, the ultimate state of being towards which yoga practice leads us. *Samadhi* is enlightenment, when, according the ancient texts, we merge into a state of blissful union with the Universe; knowing all there is to know, seeing all as it really is, with nothing left to fear. Whilst this is a lofty aim indeed, there's no doubt that we can all experience glimpses of this state of being. Maybe you've felt a sense of complete freedom and timelessness whilst gazing at an ocean, skiing down a mountain, or lying in the arms of a loved one – in a state of 'no-mind', experiencing yourself as pure Being, pure Presence, totally in the now. Can you recall a time in your life when you have felt so intimately connected to the Source? That feeling of being one with the Universe is a tiny taster of our true nature.

The first section of the Yoga Sutras is entitled *Samadhi Pada* (a *pada* in this context is a chapter).

Samadhi is described in the Yoga Sutras as complete spontaneous understanding of the object – there is no separation between the seeing, the seer and the seen as they merge into unity. There are no labels, no interpretations, only direct experience and the ultimate wisdom of direct comprehension.

There are two main states of *samadhi* – *sabija* or *samprajnata samadhi*, meaning *samadhi* 'with a seed' or 'with an object' (such as the ocean, mountain, or loved one in the above example); and *nirbija* or *asamprajnata samadhi*, meaning 'seedless' or 'objectless' samadhi. In the latter nothing external plays any part, and total unity with *Brahman* (ultimate Universal Consciousness or what you may call God) is reached. (Patanjali describes other stages of *samadhi* within these states, but these are the two main categories.)

He tells us that in the earlier stage of *samadhi*, we experience the direct perception of the spiritual light of the Self – first-hand, intuitive knowledge, beyond anything that can be learnt from a book or teacher, aligned with the divine nature of all beings and things. With this, a new kind of life dawns. When even that wisdom is detached from, so arises the ultimate, 'seedless' *samadhi*.

Chapter 11 – Yoga Practices You Might Meet

Now that we've explored the foundational philosophy of yoga with the *koshas* and the eight limbs, let's take a look at the practices which help us to integrate these teachings into our lives.

In a standard studio class you'll meet *asana*, *pranayama*, and hopefully meditation. Yoga has many more tools to offer us beyond these, and in this chapter we'll explore some practices that you might meet on your yoga journey. We'll look at:

Bandha - subtle energy locks
Drishti - gaze point
Mudra - gestures
Yoga nidra - yogic sleep
Sankalpa - highest vow – a type of affirmation
Chanting, *mantra* and *kirtan* – vocal and vibrational practices
Satsang – yogic community
Kriyas – cleansing actions

<u>Bandha</u>

The word *bandha* means lock, and it refers to a subtle energy retention. (It's helpful to think of the word 'lock' as the type that you find on a canal, to restrain water, rather than the type you find on a door.) Different *asana* and *pranayama* techniques alter the flow of energy within the body. Consider how you feel after a backbending posture: your heart rate increases and you feel exhilarated. Now contrast that with a forward fold: your pulse slows, your mind quietens and there's a sense of going inwards. That's a simple example of how our energy is affected by a posture.

The *bandhas* act like locks on a canal, retaining and containing that energy where we want it. Although we first begin to find *bandhas* using physical cues, as our awareness becomes more refined we can feel them energetically.

There are three main *bandhas* that you might hear referred to in classes, particularly if you practise Ashtanga or Vinyasa yoga, and they are:

Mula bandha – root lock

Uddiyana bandha – stomach lock
Jalandhara bandha – throat lock

Mula bandha assists with stability and creating a firm foundation. On a physical level this is useful in standing and balancing postures; energetically it relates to cutting through resistance to change and becoming stuck in our ways – it creates a sense of self-trust as we develop our own inner stability.

We can begin to locate it by squeezing the pelvic floor muscles, as though trying to stop urination mid-flow. At first it's normal to find that the whole pelvic floor area contracts, from the front of the urethra to the back of the anus. The pelvic floor is a fairly large hammock-like area of muscle which supports the contents of the pelvic bowl. With patient practice, we can begin to refine this contraction, so that we're not simply squeezing everything inwards, but finding a sense of lift; a feeling of rising up towards the navel. The next step is to locate and isolate the contraction of the three main areas within the pelvic floor: at the rear around the anus; in the middle the top of the vagina for women or perineum for men; and at the front the urethra (which is the trickiest for most people to isolate). *Mula bandha*'s closest physical location is the middle one, the vagina or perineum, and it's engagement raises the downward energy of *apana vayu* to meet the rising energy of *prana vayu*, resulting in increased vitality. (See chapter 12 for more on the *vayus*.)

It's important to use *bandhas* dynamically. A healthy muscle is not only strong but responsive and elastic, and keeping a tightly gripped pelvic floor for extended periods can have unintended consequences, especially for women, who may experience difficulty in sexual intercourse and childbirth if the muscles become tight and stiff. Paradoxically the muscles can also be weakened by constant over-engagement and create incontinence. It is inadvisable to use strong *mula bandha* when menstruating or pregnant, if constipated, or if you have an IUD fitted.

After using a lot of *mula bandha* during a long practice, I recommend rapidly 'pumping' the entire pelvic floor about twenty times to keep it responsive and flexible. Balance and moderation is key in all things, and used judiciously *bandhas* can greatly enhance one's practice both in physical stability and lightness, and energetic awareness.

It's important to use *bandhas* dynamically. A healthy muscle is not only strong but responsive and elastic, and keeping a tightly gripped pelvic floor for extended periods can have unintended consequences, especially for women, who may experience difficulty in sexual intercourse and childbirth if the muscles become tight and stiff. Paradoxically the muscles can also be weakened by constant over-engagement and create incontinence. It is inadvisable to use strong *mula bandha* when menstruating or pregnant, if constipated, or if you have an IUD fitted.

After using a lot of *mula bandha* during a long practice, I recommend rapidly 'pumping' the entire pelvic floor about twenty times to keep it responsive and flexible. Balance and moderation is key in all things, and used judiciously *bandhas* can greatly enhance one's practice both in physical stability and lightness, and energetic awareness.

Uddiyana translates as 'flying up', and it's this energetic action of the physical stomach lock which assists us in lightly jumping forward and back in sun salutations and vinyasas, and taking flight in arm balancing poses. It stretches and tones the respiratory diaphragm, and a light touch of *uddiyana bandha* can also help us to maintain a good standing posture. Energetically this *bandha* is associated with raising our energy to the higher centres, allowing us to offer our talents and work openly and generously to the world (more about this in the next chapter).

There are two main ways to use *uddiyana bandha*. The first is the full stomach lock, which is easiest to find from Downward Dog. **Make sure it's at least two hours since your last meal before trying this! An empty**

stomach is best. Having established yourself in a steady full breathing pattern in the pose, start to more fully complete your exhales so that your abdomen begins to hollow out. Allow the muscles of the abdomen to be soft and relaxed; don't try and hold your stomach in. Then, with a completed exhale and concave abdomen, make as if to inhale, but don't actually take any air in. With practice, you'll find that your abdomen fully rises up 'into' your ribcage, so that if you look back to your belly you'll see it completely hollowed out. This is the physical expression of full *uddiyana bandha*. To feel the lightness that this offers, experiment with pouncing your feet forwards to your hands, taking your bottom high into the air, as you begin your next inhale. This full vacuum effect is most commonly used in *kriyas* such as *agni sara* and *nauli* (see page 108).

The second way involves a much subtler application of the *bandha* which allows you to breathe at the same time, with the breath remaining in the thoracic region of your torso (as opposed to belly breathing). First find the full version of the *bandha*, then try engaging just 30% of it – engaging your tranverse abdominus muscle in the lower abdomen. This is a useful *uddiyana bandha* in poses where lightness and lift is required, such as *Bakasana* (crow pose).

> To find your tranverse abdominus, lie flat on your back with your legs outstretched and feet flexed as though you were standing up. Put your hands on your lower abdomen just inside your hipbones. Now, imagine you have a heavy sandbag on your legs. Reach firmly into your heels and try to lift the bag using only your legs, but pretend it's so heavy you can't move. Did you feel the muscles switch on beneath your fingers? That's your TA.

Jalandhara bandha is most commonly used when working with specific *pranayama* and breath retention (*kumbhaka*) practices. Physically, it stimulates the thyroid and parathyroid glands, and is associated with the ability to express ourselves in a responsible manner. If *mula bandha* is the base of the energy container, and *uddiyana* allows us to direct the energy held within, *jalandhara* can be thought of as the lid of the container.

To find *jalandhara bandha* we first need to make sure that our skull is correctly placed atop the spine. You might think 'where else would it be?', but it's possible and common for us to have a poor postural structure here.

As we saw earlier, the skull rests on the very top of the spine, where the uppermost vertebrae create a spigot and ring called the dens and the Atlas bone. When the skull is optimally aligned on these bones, the head is so well supported that there is minimal muscular effort required to hold it and it pivots freely, almost as though it were floating. Unfortunately modern life habits such as looking at smartphones mean that this ideal alignment becomes compromised, often resulting in neck and shoulder tension as our muscles are forced to support our heavy heads like the guyropes of a tent, under both load and tension.

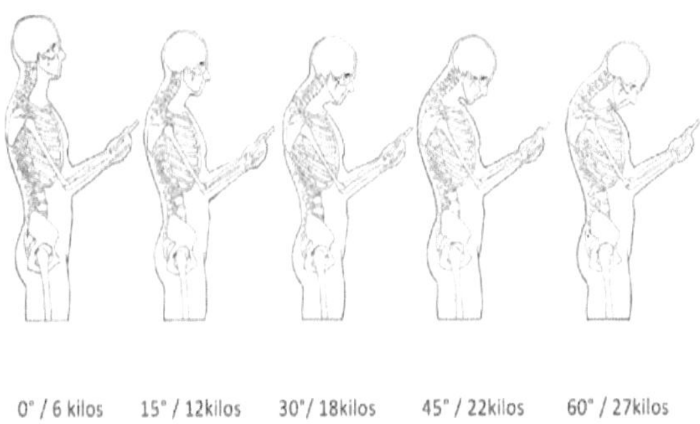

So let's find that optimum alignment.

Sit on a chair, or cross-legged on the floor, and either way have a firm cushion or folded blanket under the rear part of your buttocks so that your pelvis is slightly tilted forward. This encourages the natural lumbar curve of your spine, setting up a good chain of vertebral structure.

Now, sit tall, as though your spine is a tree growing out of the pot of your pelvis. Slightly tilt your head back; then draw your chin a little towards your sternum, as though you're trying to hold an orange in the space in front of your throat.

Visualise a skewer going through your ears. The point where the skewer would meet your spine is the location of the dens: the pivot point between your spine and skull. Now, maintaining that alignment and visualisation, slowly turn your head from side to side. If you have found the optimal alignment, your head will feel as though it is turning with minimal effort and your neck muscles will remain soft until the 60-70 degree mark, when your sternomastocledoid muscle (the one that juts out between jaw and collarbone when you turn your head) on the opposite side to the way you are turning will engage.

If this initial alignment feels very different from your usual posture it's a good idea to simply spend time working with this. This is how our heads are supposed to sit, and from here we can start to find *jalandhara bandha*.

Place your hands on your legs so that your arms are straight. Slightly retract your tongue so that the tip of it rests against the roof of your mouth where the hard and soft palates meet. Take a full breath in, and exhale fully. As you maintain the pause at the end of the exhale, lower your chin towards your sternum so that it rests against the upper part of your chest. (This is not anatomically possible for some people – if that applies to you, simply lower your chin to your neck as far as you comfortably can.) Continue to breathe here and observe how the mind becomes quieter – this is basic *jalandhara bandha*.

Our bodies are vessels for energy, and *asana* facilitates the free flow of *prana* (life-force). *Bandhas* then help us to retain energy within the container of the torso and channel its flow, just like a dam retains the power of water to be diverted for a particular use. *Bandhas* take our *asana* practice to the next level - there is far more to an *asana* than a physical shape. They are not a beginner's practice – first we must learn to breathe *dirgha sukshma* (long and smooth) and find *sthira* (steadiness) and *sukha* (ease) in the posture. Then we may learn to shape our breath (see chapter 6), and when we are proficient in these stages we are ready to add the more subtle energy work of the *bandhas*.

<u>Drishti</u>

Drishti means 'gaze point', and refers to where we focus our eyes. It is commonly used during an *asana* practice as a way of harnessing our mental attention and improving concentration, as well as making more complex poses easier or harder. For example, try standing in Tree pose and looking around wildly. How easy is it to balance? Can you regulate your breathing? How likely is it that you could quieten your thoughts like this?

Now, find a fixed point straight in front of you to gaze at. Notice how your breathing becomes more regular, your mind settles, and how your balance stabilises. Then slowly move your gaze upwards towards the sky, as though tracing an invisible vertical line with your eyes. What effect does that have on your balance? You may start to sway and wobble, maybe fall out of the pose. And finally, try closing your eyes – balancing suddenly becomes very challenging indeed!

Different poses traditionally have different *drishti*; for example, in *Virabhadrasana I* (Warrior 1) the gaze is to the thumbs; *Virabhadrasana II* (Warrior 2) takes it over the middle finger of the forward hand; and *Virabhadrasana III* (Warrior 3) moves it about to the floor about a metre in front of your head.

Engaging a *drishti* is a form of *pratyahara* (sense withdrawal) and *dharana* (concentration). Our energy or *prana* goes in the direction of our attention; so it follows that if we are distracted in an *asana* and looking around the room, our *prana* is also scattered. By gazing softly at a fixed point we withdraw our minds from the distractions of the visual world and concentrate our attention, and so contain and direct our *prana*.

<u>*Mudra*</u>

Mudra refers to a gesture or hand position. You're probably familiar with at least two *mudras*: *jnana mudra*, where the thumb and index finger are brought to touch with the palms upturned and (often) resting on the thighs in a seated position; and *anjali mudra*, or prayer position with the palms together in front of the centre of the chest.

The purpose of mudra on a gross level is to focus the concentration; and more subtly, to channel the flow of *prana* within the body. Whilst it takes time and practice to refine the awareness to a degree where we can FEEL this energy shift, the shift happens even if we're not able to feel it yet.

There is also a mind-body connection element to working with *mudras*. Just like with *drishti*, energy goes in the direction of our attention. When we place our hands in a particular *mudra* with the intention of bringing about a related effect, it plants a seed in the subconscious and works powerfully with the placebo effect of the brain to bring about tangible results.

We all use gestures in everyday life as part of our body language, and the languages of some nationalities are well-known for involving extensive and enthusiastic gesturing. Think of the gestures that say 'I don't know'; 'thank you'; 'hello'; 'that one'; and 'stop', without words. Mudras are an extension of that – some have more subtle effects than others, but all work with our mind-body connection and movements of energy within our bodies to elicit a specific effect.

Here are a couple of experiments with *mudra* for you to try – with very little practice, many people can feel the effects of these.

Experiment 1 - *Sharira mudras*

Sharira means 'body', and the *sharira mudras* are placements of our hands on different areas of the torso to help facilitate changes in breathing. We'll work with three body areas here: belly, ribs and chest.

Firstly try breathing into only your lower abdomen for a few breaths. Then see if you can breathe only into your side ribs. Thirdly, try breathing only into your chest.

Now repeat the process with the addition of the following *Sharira mudras* and see if you experience it any differently.

1 - Sitting upright, place your hands on your lower abdomen with thumb tips touching each other just below your navel, and index fingers meeting to form a triangle shaped gap between your hands. Now, breathe 'into' your hands, feeling the area below them inflate and deflate like a balloon. Stay with this for ten full, deep breaths.

2 - Now, move your hands up to your ribcage, midway between your nipples and navel. Place your thumbs pointing to the rear of your body and lift your palms away from your ribs, so that only the 'L' shape formed by the inside edges of your thumbs and forefingers rest against the sides of your ribs.

Breathe 'into' those points of contact and see how much you can make your ribs flare up and out with your breath (a useful visual is the movement of an umbrella as it opens). Stay for ten breaths.

3 - Next, keep the shape of your hands as they are and slide them up the sides of your body about six inches, so that your index fingers are just above your nipple line and your thumbs are in your lower armpits. How much movement can you create there, in an 'up and out' movement towards your outer shoulders, using only your breath?

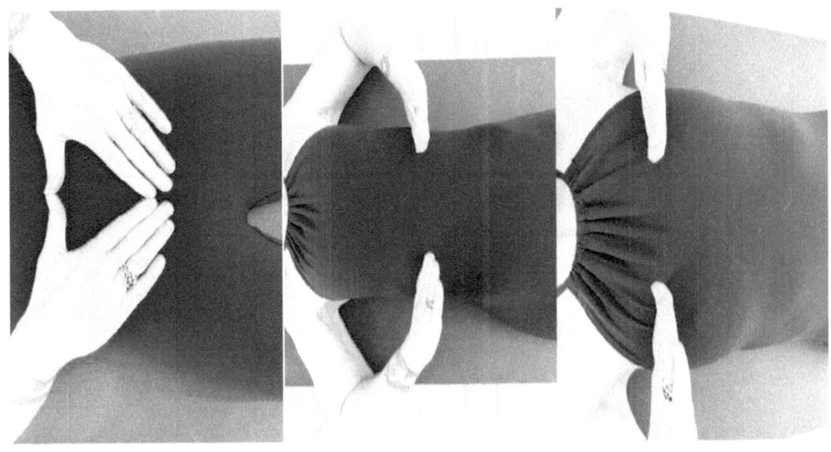

How did your experience differ, with and without hands? Was it easier to 'find' your breath with the mind-body connection established by the *mudras*?

Experiment 2 – *Merundanda mudras*

This practice is a little subtler than the previous one, but you may still be surprised by its effects.

Sit upright, either in a chair with your feet planted flat and hip width apart on the floor, or cross-legged on the floor with the rear of your pelvis elevated on a cushion.

Make 'thumbs-up' shapes with both hands, as though you're hitchhiking.

Position 1 – Place your hands on your knees or thighs with your fingernails against your legs and the thumbs pointing in towards each other. Close your eyes, breathe deeply, and notice where you feel your breath most fully.

Position 2 – Keep the hand position and turn your fists so your thumbs are pointing to the sky. Turn your attention inwards, breathe deeply, and notice where you feel your breath now.

Position 3 – Maintain the same hand position and turn your fists so the backs of your hands are against your legs and the thumbs are pointing out, away from each other. Again, notice where you feel your breath most keenly now.

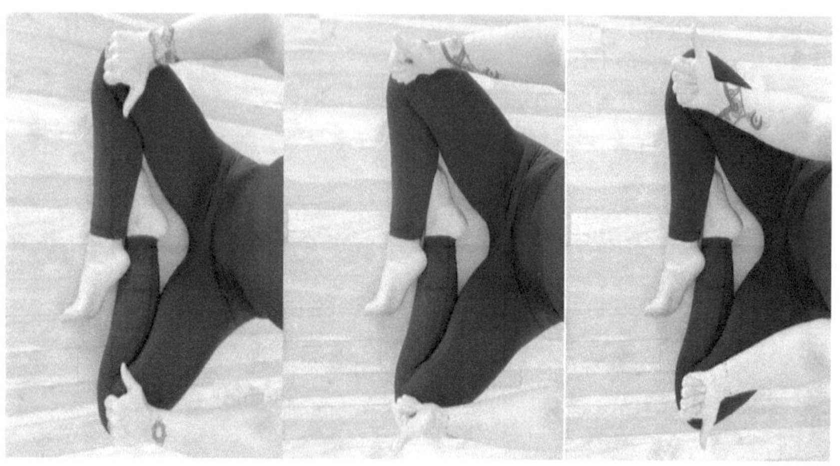

Could you feel a difference between the three positions?

With practice and attention, you'll notice that your breath 'climbs' up your body with each position. In 1, most of the breath is felt in the lower abdomen. In 2, the ribs; and in 3, the chest. The change happens partly because of the way the shape of your torso alters slightly with each position, which in turn alters the space around the lungs and spine, and therefore the way in which *prana* (energy/the life-force) moves (see chapter 12 for more on *prana*). If you didn't feel it the first time, try again now and play around with it.

There are a vast number of *mudras* to bring about different effects within us. Most of them are more subtle than the two we just experimented with, but with time and practice you'll begin to refine your interoceptive awareness and begin to notice subtle shifts in how you feel when you use them.

Here are some *mudras* you might meet.

Anjali mudra

Probably the most familiar of all *mudras*, the gesture of palms pressed together ('prayer hands' or '*namaste* hands') signifies recognition, gratitude or reverence.

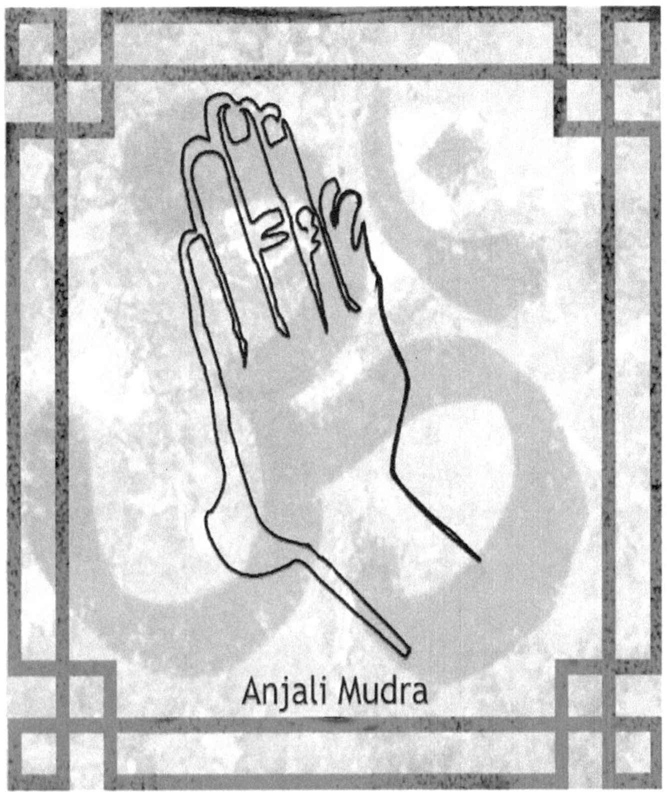

Jnana mudra

Another familiar gesture, in *jnana mudra* we bring the thumbtip and index fingertip together with the palms facing up. The thumb represents the Universal Consciousness, the finger our individual nature, and in joining them together we recognise that we are part of a greater whole. The palms face upwards to signify receptivity to greater awareness and understanding; true knowledge and wisdom or *jnana*.

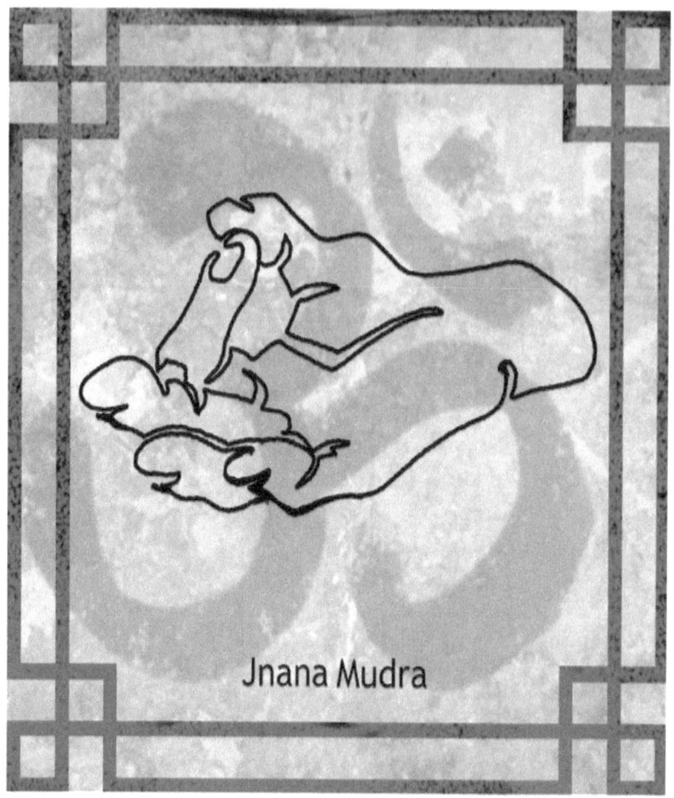

<u>*Chin mudra*</u>

In *chin mudra* the thumb and forefinger are in the same arrangement as *jnana mudra*, but the palms face downwards. This is a gesture of learning, humility, and wisdom.

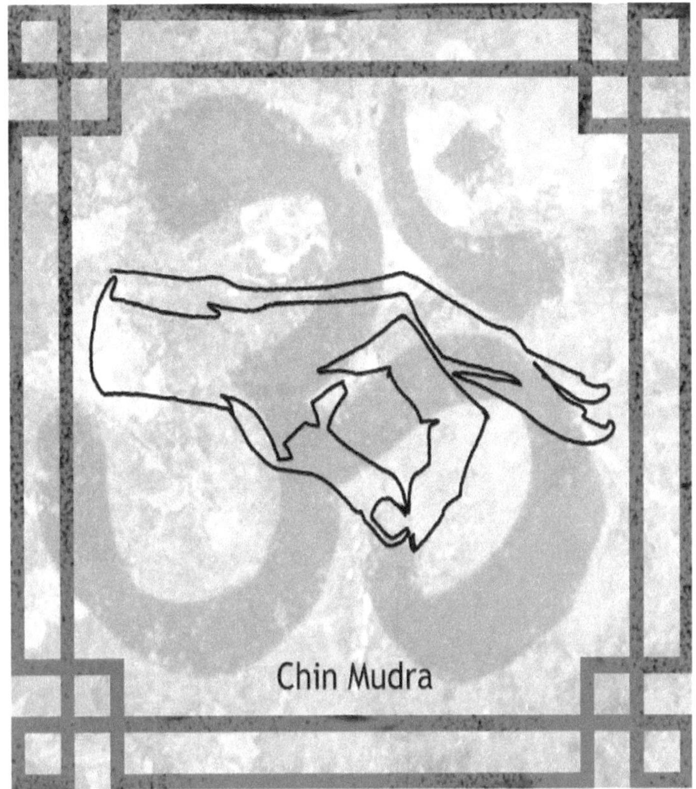

Yoni mudra

Yoni is the Sanskrit term for the female reproductive system. In *yoni mudra*, the thumb tips touch each other, and the index fingertips meet so that the hands form an upside-down triangle. The other fingers can be tucked back into the palms as a 'free-standing' mudra; alternatively this can be practised with the hands on the lower belly and the thumbs resting below the navel just as in the *Sharira mudras*. This *mudra* represents the feminine or *'Shakti'* energy (which men have too – we are all a blend of the masculine and feminine forces in differing quantities). As you've experienced, this is a very useful *mudra* to help us to connect with belly breathing, and can also used as a therapeutic tool for bringing awareness and energy to the *yoni* area.

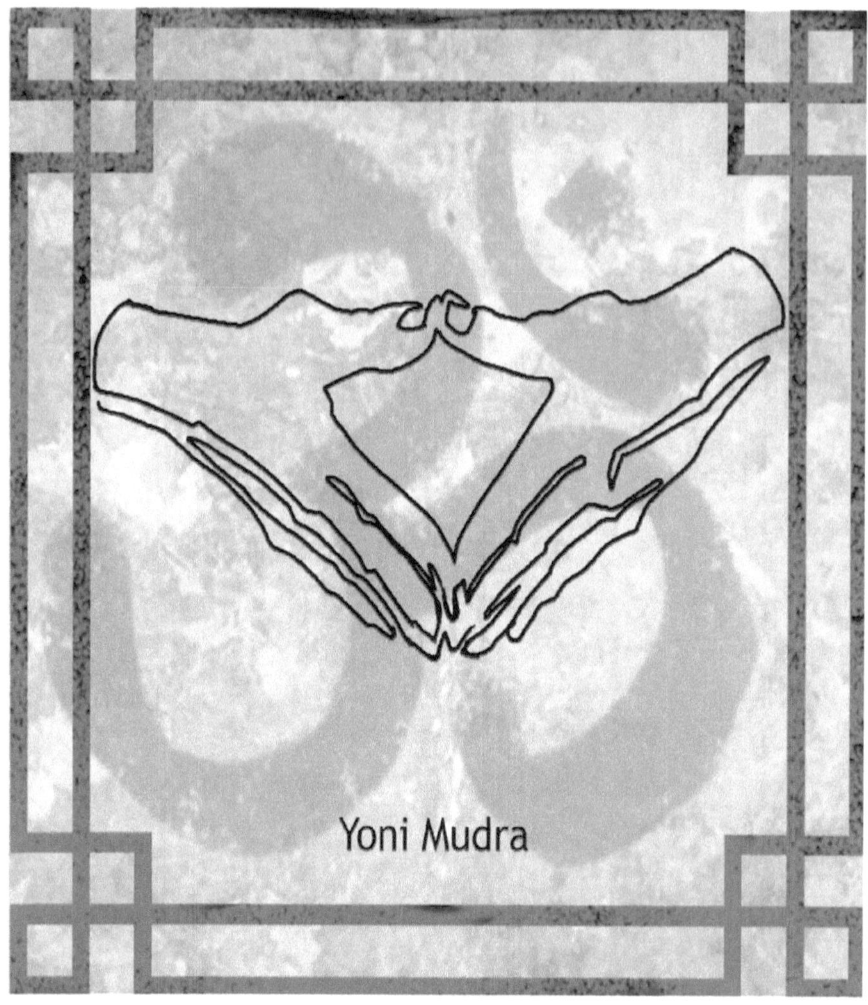

Yoga Nidra

Yoga Nidra, meaning 'yogic sleep', is a state of consciousness. The practice, which has its roots in Tantra (see chapter 17), is a form of *pratyahara* – all of the senses are withdrawn except for hearing as we enter a kind of dynamic sleep – the body and mind rest, whilst a deeper level of consciousness remains aware.

During *yoga nidra* we experience a very deep form of guided relaxation in which, despite the name, we stay awake. Through a series of steps such as moving the awareness around many points of the body, visualisation, and considering pairs of opposite feelings, we take the consciousness into the slowest delta brain-wave state which is usually only found during the deepest part of the sleep cycle, but we remain awake and aware. We surf a liminal state between waking and sleep, on the threshold of the conscious and subconscious mind, and the practice is profoundly restorative as this is the state in which the body and brain do extremely effective repair work. Through the stages of *yoga nidra*, the body and brain are guided to release stored tension and fully relax. You may think 'surely sleep does that', but it's entirely possible – and common - to fall asleep in a tense state when we're under stress, and wake up feeling exhausted. For this reason it's sometimes said that an hour of *yoga nidra* is as effective as four hours of sleep; and whilst *yoga nidra* should not be used as a replacement for normal sleep, a twenty or thirty minute practice is a fabulous afternoon pick-me-up which shifts us into the parasympathetic relaxation response of the nervous system (which we explored in chapter 6).

Yoga nidra is far more than a pleasant guided relaxation, it's a powerful tool for profound insight and transformation. The process moves us from the normal waking beta brain wave state (12.5 – 30 cycles per second), down through the more relaxed alpha state (8-12 cycles per second), and then into a theta state (4-8 cycles) where creativity and inspiration are greatly enhanced. But we're just passing through even that, on the way to a delta state where brain waves are very slow, just 0.5 – 4 cycles per second.

In this hypnagogic delta state we experience a loosening of ego-identifications, and increased openness, sensitivity, and empathy. Creativity and attention-span increases and heart rate variability improves. Insufficient time spent in the delta brain wave state is associated with depression and anxiety; it is in this state that the brain chemical dopamine, which is responsible for feelings of motivation, is produced.

Yoga and brain chemistry

We know that practising yoga makes us feel good, but why?

Dopamine – the motivating one. Increases social behaviour, improves concentration, is released in pleasurable situations to motivate us to repeat them. As we've just seen, dopamine is boosted by the deeply relaxed state induced by *yoga nidra*.

Serotonin – the happy one. Elevates mood, reduces aggression, increases resistance to anxiety and depression. Yoga indirectly affects serotonin production by promoting relaxation and feelings of overall wellbeing, and improving sleep. Adequate sleep is vital to serotonin production.

Oxytocin – the loved-up one. Promotes feelings of trust, empathy, affection and bonding. Increased oxytocin levels have been noted in meditators and people practising gratitude.

Endorphin – the high-on-life one. Creates a sense of well being and even euphoria, relieves pain, reduces stress. Physical exercise, including yoga *asana*, stimulates the circulation of endorphins.

GABA – the relaxing one. Relieves anxiety, elevates mood, helps induce sleep. Yoga's relaxing effect on the nervous system helps with balancing GABA.

Cortisol and adrenalin – the stressy ones. These vital chemicals are our bodies' natural defence mechanisms in times of stress and danger, and are literally lifesavers in acute situations (see chapter 6). However, many of us live with high levels of stress and these chemicals become chronically elevated, causing harm. The rebalancing effect of yoga on the nervous system helps to being them back into a healthy state.

So what actually happens during *yoga nidra*? Well, externally, not much! All you do is lie down, use whatever props you like to get really comfortable, close your eyes, and follow the verbal guidance. This is not a *dharana* (concentration) practice, and you don't intensely focus on the guidance – you just let it wash over you and follow the words. At first it's quite common to fall asleep during the practice, and although the idea is to stay aware, it's not a big deal or a waste of time if you sleep - your subconscious will still receive some benefit as by that stage it will be deeply relaxed. Ultimately though, the idea is to consciously experience the deeper layers of our psyche, of which we're usually only aware for the briefest moment before falling into a dream state. The practice opens this channel and offers a unique opportunity to connect with our innermost self and receive its intuitive guidance.

Yoga nidra is therefore a powerful means by which to facilitate self-healing, connect with our own intuition and inner wisdom, and empower ourselves.

In this deeply relaxed state, the subconscious and unconscious mind are very receptive to impressions placed in them. This may sound like hypnosis, but it is different. We may pass through a state of hypnosis, but we quickly go beyond it as we retract attention from all external stimuli except the auditory channel whilst remaining conscious. Hypnosis is a dull, *tamasic*, closed-down state; *yoga nidra* is an enlivened, *sattvic*, open and receptive state (see chapter 16 for full definitions of *tamasic* and *sattvic*). If I lead you into *yoga nidra*, there is no way that I can make you do anything such as eat a raw onion or dance a jig – you are the one who is in control at all times because you are conscious and you are following the instruc**tions** not the instruct**or**. All of the 'instructions' are offered suggestions, and only you can choose to bring about changes – you are **consciously** functioning at a very deep level.

The stages of *yoga nidra* are as follows:

1 - Settling in
2 – *Sankalpa*
3 – Breath awareness
4 – Rotation of consciousness
5 – Breath awareness
6 – Pairs of opposites
7 – Counting

8 – Visualisation
9 – *Sankalpa*
10 – Return to waking state

However, it's not mandatory to include all of these stages. The stages in bold type are the stages which must be present, the rest are optional (but generally remain in the same place in the order). As this gives a lot of scope for a tailored practice, *yoga nidra* can vary greatly in duration – it may be as brief as twelve to fifteen minutes, or as long as an hour.

To expand upon the stages:

1 – Settling in. You get comfortable, make any final adjustments so that you can remain motionless throughout the practice, and tell yourself that you are practising *yoga nidra* and will remain awake and aware.

2 – *Sankalpa*. This means 'highest vow', and is a resolve, or a statement of intention. The word '*san*' refers to a connection with our highest truth, and '*kalpa*' means vow. So a *sankalpa* is a commitment to our highest truth and most heartfelt desires; a statement to which you can continually return, to guide your choices and remind yourself of your true nature and purpose. It comes from the premise that you are already who you need to be in order to fulfil your *dharma* or life's purpose, and all you need to do is connect to your most heartfelt desires, focus your mind, and channel the energy within.

In *yoga nidra* you may be invited to repeat your *sankalpa* silently to yourself at certain points. The effect of this statement, crafted to speak to your subconscious in its own language, at a time when it is in its most deeply relaxed and receptive state, is profound and offers incredible potential in transforming life patterns. It can be used to guide the subconscious and unconscious mind to accomplish almost anything.

3 – Breath awareness. You are invited to witness the effortless flow of breath in and out of your body.

4 – Rotation of consciousness. You go on a journey of awareness around many different points of your body. In a fascinating demonstration of the power of directed awareness, volunteers were connected up to brain scanning equipment during this process. In the same way as you'd expect to see a particular area of the brain activate in response to the corresponding body

part being touched, so it was when mental awareness was placed there with no touch. This rotation of consciousness takes you progressively deeper into sense withdrawal and a meditative state.

5 – Breath awareness. Step 3 is repeated.

6 – Pairs of opposites. You are invited to imagine different sensations, as though you are actually feeling them, for example, heaviness then lightness; cold then warmth. Then you may be invited to let them co-exist simultaneously. This has the effect of temporarily 'short-circuiting' the analytical, reasoning part of the brain which says that two opposing things cannot exist together, and takes you into a state of non-dual awareness, that everything simply is as it is and all is one. (This is a very Tantrik perspective on life.) Repeated practice allows simultaneous nerve operation between different parts of the brain and establishes new neural connections. This is a very empowering part of the practice, because you have the direct experience that your consciousness can direct your experience of sensations rather than you being at their mercy.

In more advanced *yoga nidra* practices, you may be invited to experience opposing emotions. This is a part of the practice that a guide must approach with caution, as it has the potential to bring up repressed trauma - practitioners are in a vulnerable state and placing their trust in the guide. If you are planning to teach *yoga nidra*, I would recommend a policy of 'if in doubt, don't' for this part, especially in a group setting where you may not know the people well. In my opinion this is a technique best left to one-on-one practice, with a very experienced guide working with a client with whom the therapeutic relationship is already well established. With such caution heeded however, this is a profoundly valuable practice in developing the potential to go beyond judgment and duality, resulting in emotional stability and the capacity to overcome unhelpful reactions and consciously direct one's own life.

7 – Counting. You are invited to count your breaths down from a specific number, usually a factor of the sacred number 108, thereby further withdrawing consciousness from external stimulation.

8 – Visualisation. By now you are deeply into a liminal state of awareness. You are asked to be aware of the 'movie screen' of your awareness and conjure a scene, or a variety of different images. This both develops the ability to witness events with non-attachment, and increases the communication between the waking and dream states. Our dreams have valuable messages from our intuition for us, and this part of the practice cultivates improved access to *vijnanamaya kosha*.

9 – *Sankalpa.* With the subconscious and unconscious mind now in a deeply relaxed and receptive state, like a fertile field that has been carefully prepared

for planting, you once again sow the seed of your *sankalpa*.

10 – Return to waking state. The guide invites you to re-establish awareness of your body and surroundings, and gradually return to wakefulness.

In a state of *yoga nidra*, there is a sense of deep peace and freedom. It goes far beyond other types of guided relaxation. Whilst it's common to encounter *yoga nidra* being read from a standard script, this is a deep practice and script-reading can feel inert and lack the energy and nuance of a tailored, spontaneously delivered practice.

Advanced practitioners may be able to guide themselves into *yoga nidra* – and it can certainly be valuable to use elements of the practice as stand-alone enhancements to everyday life. For example, doing a rotation of consciousness around your body is a great way to calm yourself when stressed or help you to get to sleep at night; and repeating your *sankalpa* to yourself helps to strengthen its effects.

Sankalpa

Finding our true purpose is no mean feat! *Sankalpa* is really always one thing - a call to awakening. But to realise the deepest aspect of our own *sankalpa*, we may have to go through some stages along the way, like stepping stones across a river, each step within reach of the previous and next ones. In this way, *sankalpa* can be used for both therapeutic purposes and higher purposes (such as Self-realisation).

The stages could be said to be:

a - Changing unhelpful habits
b - Improving quality of life
c - Creating a genuine change within the personality
d - Realising true purpose

We word a *sankalpa* by using positive statements in the present tense, as though it is already happening - this is a powerful technique which works with the subconscious mind. Our subconscious minds do not readily process negation words such as 'no' and 'not'; so when we say 'I'm **not** going to do x', the subconscious doesn't respond to the '**not**'. In effect we therefore program ourselves to do the exact opposite of what we're trying to achieve –

no wonder New Year's resolutions don't work! Using negation words also gives the conscious mind something to argue with – I don't know about you, but the fastest way to make me do something is to tell me I'm not to do it! Using positive statements – telling me what you **do** want me to do – is far more likely to be effective.

Using the present tense is in line with the premise that we are already all we need to be, and that change can be effected in every moment – no need to put it off, because NOW is the only time that anything can ever happen!

For example, you might decide that you would like to be more patient and understanding with your loved ones. Your *sankalpa* could be 'compassion is my true nature'. Or you may decide that you want to improve your health by eating better - your *sankalpa* might be 'I nourish my body with fresh healthy food'. Or perhaps you feel unfulfilled and are struggling to find what you really want to do with your life. Your *sankalpa* may be 'I connect with my deepest desires and trust my instincts'.

A properly worded *sankalpa* follows these guidelines:

Positive statements - ie instead of 'I will not smoke', try 'I breathe clean fresh air'.

Present tense: ie instead of 'I will achieve my dreams', try 'I apply myself fully to achieving my dreams', or even simply 'I achieve my dreams'.

Significant: don't waste your *sankalpa* on material things. However, if you feel something is lacking in your life, you might say 'I receive limitless abundance and opportunity'.

Personal: we can only change our own behaviour and reactions.

Flexible enough to account for changing circumstances.

Whilst the above examples would not be regarded as statements of ultimate life purpose, they form the stepping stones to move us in that direction.

Chanting, *Mantra* and *Kirtan*

Chanting

In ancient India where literacy was uncommon, the wisdom of the Vedas, Yoga Sutras, and other sacred texts was passed from teacher to student by chanting. The language of Sanskrit has vibrational qualities which are unparalleled by modern language, and learning through the medium of chanting brings the verses to life in a way which reading does not, as well as helping us commit them to memory. Chanting is not like singing – only a few tones are used, and the sound produced tends to be more throaty and guttural than song.

Mantra

A *mantra* is a sacred sound which produces a particular energetic effect through vibration. In the Tantrik tradition they are representations of deities in vibrational form, and can be chanted aloud or mentally. The word mantra is derived from '*man*' – mind – and '*tra*' – to protect and liberate. *Mantras* were revealed in deep meditation to the ancient yogis.

Traditional *mantras* are given in the same Sanskrit language that we hear in the names of *yoga asana*. Mysterious, complex and beautiful, Sanskrit originated in India around 3,500 years ago. Sound is a representation of the Universe itself - because all sound is vibration - and all the matter of the Universe is made up of vibration of energy. Correct pronunciation and tonal nuance is extremely important in Sanskrit – sacred sound was an important part of the search for spiritual liberation. Language is our primary way of communicating ideas and inspiration, and spoken Sanskrit was believed to be a perfect language, containing special powers within the weight of its syllables.

Many *mantras*, particularly those from the Tantrik tradition, are secret and must be passed from teacher to student in an initiation ceremony. Other universal *mantras* may be used by anyone. Examples are '*Om*' (the sound of the Universal Consciousness itself), '*so ham*' (the sound of the breath, also meaning 'I am That' ie a microcosm of the Universe); the *bija* seed mantras which correspond with the *chakras* (*lam, vam, ram, yam, ham, Om*); and the longer verse of the beautiful *Gayatri mantra*.

From a physical perspective, chanting a *mantra* has the effect of lengthening exhalation (try it for yourself with an '*Om*'), thereby calming the nervous system. Mentally, the concentration required quietens mind chatter.

Energetically, the vibration of chanting stimulates the hypothalamus in the brain, an important fuction of which is linking the nervous system with the endocrine system via the pituitary gland, which is associated with the third eye chakra (see next chapter).

A common way to practise with a *mantra* is to count *japa* (repetitions). Counting the repetitions off using *mala* beads is a useful way to keep track – you might choose to do a whole *mala* (108 repetitions), or fold the *mala* in half or quarter to measure out 54 or 27 repetitions of the *mantra*. Then you might sit in silence and mentally repeat the *mantra* without counting, and watch how your mind and awareness respond. Remain aware of the meaning of your *mantra* so there is an enlivened quality to it, rather than letting the repetition become mechanical.

<u>*Kirtan*</u>

Kirtan is chanting combined with music and shared in a group. Typically at a *kirtan* session participants sit in a circle, and the person or people leading the session may have instruments such as a harmonium, acoustic guitar and various pieces of percussion. Those leading the group might chant each line in Sanskrit, followed by the group, call and response style, so that everyone can become familiar with the whole chant. With that established, the whole group will then chant the *mantra* together, many times over, sometimes louder, sometimes quieter. This has all the effects of solo chanting, enhanced by the palpable group energy (which can be physically felt flowing in a particular direction within the circle – it's common to feel yourself spontaneously sway!), the creativity of the music, and the sense of belonging which comes from being with others. Humans are social animals, and this kind of group bonding releases the feelgood chemical of oxytocin in the brain, and also dials down the limbic system (the primitive part of the brain involved in fight/flight response). As a chant draws to a close, we generally sit in meditative silence for a period of time, enjoying the sense of inner stillness and the uplifting vibration of the raised group energy.

<u>*Satsang*</u>

Group chanting and *kirtan* are themselves a form of *satsang*, meaning a spiritual discourse or sacred gathering (*sat* = true, *sang* = association or company). We come together in a group to share and discuss ideas of spirituality. This might take the form of a talk by a teacher followed by group discussion, or there might be a chosen topic and each person will offer their thoughts on it. *Satsang* is a beautiful way to connect with like-minded individuals and deepen our understanding.

We can also practise inner *satsang*, which seeks to raise our consciousness to a level where we realise that our individual soul

(*atma*) and the Universal Consciousness (*paramatma*) are one, which is the ultimate purpose of yoga. Meditation is a form of inner *satsang*.

Kriyas

The *kriyas or shatkarma* are a series of six groups of *Hatha* yoga practices outlined in the texts the *Hatha Yoga Pradipika* and the *Gheranda Samhita*, aimed at cleansing and purifying the physical body in order to make it a suitable dwelling place for the soul. Whilst some forms of them such as *jala neti* (cleansing the nostrils with saline solution) are still practised fairly commonly today, others such as *vaso dhauti* (swallowing a length of fabric into the stomach, churning it around and then pulling it out) have largely fallen out of use. Whilst there's great value in maintaining our bodies in temple-like condition, these practices were conceived of at a time when knowledge of bio-mechanics was very limited, and so some of them may not be of as much practical use as was once believed – some can certainly seem extreme and even dangerous to a modern western understanding!

Here I'll briefly explain the ones which you are still likely to encounter today. If further investigation into the more obscure practices interests you, you'll find them in the aforementioned texts.

Dhauti

The first *kriya* is *dhauti* or body cleansing. The practice in this category which is still in common use is **agni sara** (exhaling totally before drawing the empty stomach into full *uddiyana bandha* and releasing and contracting numerous times).

Basti

Basti is rectal / intestinal cleansing. This traditionally involved sucking water into the lower intestine through the anus whilst standing in a river - the modern form of this is **enema** or **colonic irrigation**.

<u>*Neti*</u>

Neti is nasal cleansing. *Jala neti* is a nasal wash. A ***neti* pot** or *lota* is a small container with a spout – it looks like a tiny teapot. The idea is to fill the pot with a saline solution and then pour this into one nostril and allow it to flow out of the other. This is reasonably common in yoga circles today and many people find it a useful aid in managing nasal allergies as well as cleansing the nose from dusty or dirty environments.

<u>*Trataka*</u>

Trataka is **concentrated gazing**, which cleanses the eyes by making them water.

To practise, we gaze steadily at an object such as a candle flame, *mandala* or *yantra* (see chapter 20). With the object placed around a metre in front of us at chest height, we soften the eyes and focus our gaze upon it. When the eyes start to water or we feel the urge to blink, we slowly close them. There may be an image of the gaze-object on the inside of our lids; if so, we wait until the image subsides before slowly re-opening the eyes and repeating the process. If there's no image, we simply wait for a few breaths before re-opening. This is repeated for up to 10 minutes before closing the eyes and sitting in silent meditation.

Trataka brings about several results. Candle-gazing affects the pineal gland in the brain which produces the sleep-regulating hormone melatonin, making it a perfect bedtime practice and very useful in treating insomnia and jet-lag. Consider our cave-dwelling ancestors; the hypnotic and calming effect of staring into fire is one of the oldest forms of meditation known to man! Gazing at a *mandala* or *yantra* is also calming but has a different purpose – these images may have their own meaning or metaphor, and so we absorb this by sitting in quiet contemplation with the representation. The effect of *trataka* of making the eyes water can also be useful in dusty environments.

<u>*Nauli*</u>

This is the practice of **abdominal churning**, which massages the internal organs. It is generally practised in the early morning when the stomach is empty, and proficiency in *uddiyana bandha* and *agnisara* is necessary before attempting *nauli*. There are three positions: *vama* (left), *dakshina* (right) and *madhyana* (central). We begin by standing with feet wider than hip distance, knees slightly bent, and hands on knees. The stomach is then hollowed out by performing full *uddiyana bandha*, and we move the ribcage to one side. This isolates the rectus abdominus muscles on that side which become visible as a thick band of muscles. When the ribcage is moved to the other side, the muscles 'move' with it. The muscles are then rolled side to side, to create the rippling, churning effect. *Nauli* can be very useful in maintaining regular bowel habits.

Kapalbhati

Kapalbhati is most commonly known as a breathing technique whereby we take a full inhale through the nostrils, and then rapidly pump the stomach, using the muscular contraction of rectus abdominus to pull the abdomen towards the spine and so force air out through the nostrils as short, fast exhales. After each pumped exhale, there is a short, passive inhale. This technique is said to awaken and invigorate the whole brain, especially the areas responsible for subtle perception – for this reason it is sometimes called 'skull-shining breath'. It should be noted that although it is often described as a *pranayama*, it is actually a *kriya*.

The kriya practice forms described here of **agni sara, colonic irrigation, neti, trataka, nauli** and **kapalbhati** can all be beneficial to overall health when learnt from an experienced practitioner.

As we've seen in this chapter, there are a great many yoga practices beyond postures, breathwork and meditation. In chapter 17 we will explore how we can use these various techniques to enhance our personal experience of life.

*P*rana is the life force which animates us all. It is this force which is the difference between a living body and a dead one; which gives every cell in our bodies life; and which makes plants grow. It is the energy of the Universe itself, the *prana-shakti*.

Our *prana* moves along channels known as *nadis in the* subtle energy body (*pranamaya kosha*, which we met in chapter 1). There are said to be between 72,000 (according to the *Hatha Yoga Pradipika* text) and 350,000 (according to the *Shiva Samhita* text) *nadis*, and they are similar to the *qi* meridians in Chinese medicine and acupuncture. In the physical body the *nadis* correspond with the internal highways of the cardiovascular, nervous and lymphatic systems where *prana* flows in bodily fluids in the form of oxygen, nutrients, and the electrical messages between nerve cells. In the energy body, the *nadis* carry *prana*.

There are three main *nadis* which travel along the spine, called *sushumna*, *ida* and *pingala*. In the physical dimension they correspond with the spinal cord. Think for a moment about what your spinal cord does: it carries billions of neural messages in the form of tiny electrical impulses between nerve cells with the help of neurotransmitter chemicals. What are these messages, if not pure energy?

Sushumna is the central of the three energy channels; *ida* and *pingala* run alongside it and cross over each other at each *chakra* from the root *chakra* at the base of the spine, up to the third eye *chakra*.

Ida and *pingala* are like the positive and negative wires of an electrical circuit. *Ida* is the negative, which corresponds with the left nostril and the relaxation response of the parasympathetic nervous system. It is related to lunar energy qualities like coolness, intuition, passivity, introspection and creativity. These are all attributes of the right cerebral hemisphere of our brains (which controls the left side of our bodies and vice versa). *Pingala* is the positive 'wire', which corresponds with the right nostril and the readiness / fight or flight response of the sympathetic nervous system. It is related to solar energy qualities like heat, logic, action, analysis and objectivity, which are attributes of the left cerebral hemisphere.

Although we constantly use both sides of our brains, the left hemisphere is more concerned with logical, analytical functions, and the right is more to do with emotive and empathic responses.

> To explore the fascinating phenomenon of our two-sided brains, I highly recommend Dr Jill Bolte-Taylor's autobiographical book 'My Stroke of Insight', on which she also gave a TED talk. Dr Bolte-Taylor is a neuroscientist who had a massive stroke on the left side of her brain and remained lucid enough to document the process, as she observed her analytical left hemisphere go offline and she began to experience life from the expansive awareness of her right hemisphere.

Ida = right brain / left nostril and body
Pingala = left brain / right nostril and body

Nadi shodhana pranayama (alternate nostril breathing) is a method of bringing the two sides of the nervous system into balance. It's normal to experience one nostril as clearer than the other – they generally switch sides every forty minutes or so. If we're feeling lethargic, closing off the left nostril and breathing through only the right is a way to rouse ourselves. Similarly if we're feeling agitated, left nostril breathing can help to calm us down.

Sushumna nadi is the central channel – the 'sacred stream' - along which the spiritual force of *kundalini* energy flows when awakened.

The Chakras

The first mention of the *chakras* is found in the *Rig Veda*, the oldest known Sanskrit Vedic text, believed to date back to around 1700 BCE.

The central energy channel of *sushumna* is where we find them. *Chakra* means wheel, and they are energy centres which are like roundabouts on the *sushumna* highway. On a gross level they roughly correspond with the physical nerve plexuses along the spinal cord.

Nadis and Chakras

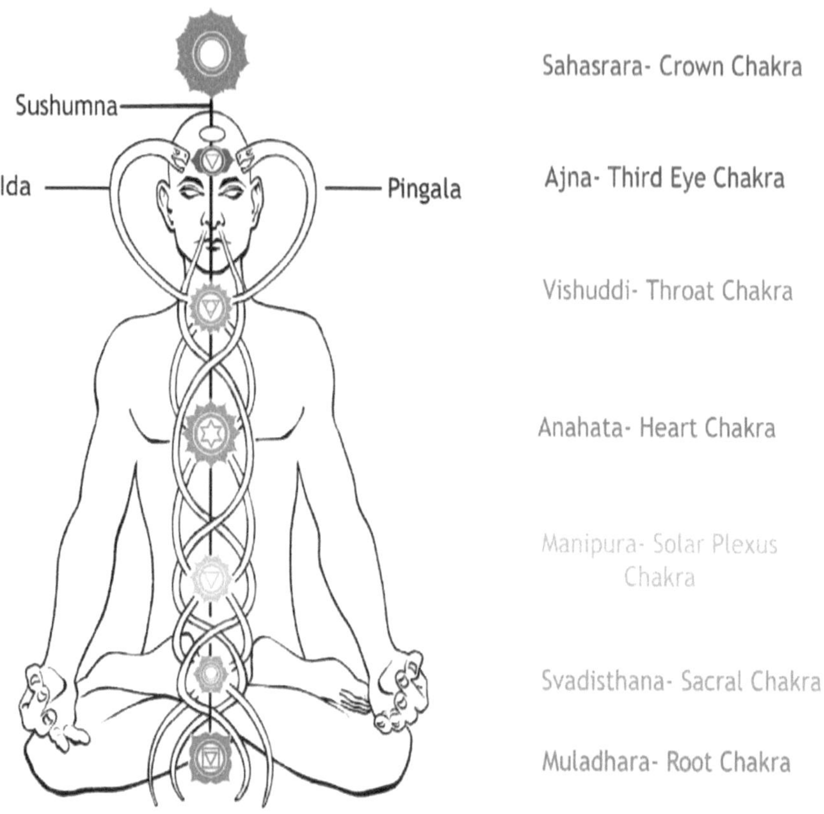

There are seven main *chakras* in the subtle energy body, from the base of the spine to slightly above the top of the head.

Each *chakra* describes a way in which we use our energy - such as feeling grounded, or creative, or motivated, or loving - and how we handle life's many circumstances. They are also associated with different areas and functions of the physical body. It's common to hear yogis speak about *chakras* being open, but it might be more accurate to say that rather than a *chakra* being open or closed like a door, all *chakras* are in play at all times and we can be in a state of deficiency, excess or balance in each one as a result of our individual psychology, self-beliefs, behaviours and life situations. Deficiency in a particular *chakra* means that we have difficulty in embodying that *chakra*'s characteristics in our life. An excess of energy in a *chakra* manifests as an over-amplification of those qualities in the related areas. For example, someone who has spent a lot of their life moving from place to place may feel perpetually anxious and unsettled, even unsafe. That would be a deficiency in *muladhara* (root*)* *chakra*, which describes feelings of stability, survival, and security. Conversely, someone who has overly absorbed western society's 'bigger, better, faster, more' message may feel compelled to try and prove their worth by aggressively pushing themselves and their employees to a state of burnout with their disproportionate drive and ambition. That would be an excess of energy in *manipura* (solar plexus) *chakra*, which describes assertiveness, personal power, and manifesting one's will in the world.

When there is balance in each *chakra*, we live our lives in a state of harmony – energy is appropriately distributed and there is neither too much nor too little energy in each area. The practices and philosophy of yoga can help us to work holistically with our own needs to bring us closer to a state of equilibrium. Generally speaking, if there was deficiency in a particular area, you would adopt the suggested practices for that area; if there was an excess, you may work with increasing energy in the *chakras* either side of it.

If you recognise your own tendencies within the following descriptions, you may find it helpful to incorporate the associated suggested practices into your life. However this is a general guide for mild imbalances and cannot replace the more in-depth help provided by working closely with an experienced teacher or yoga therapist. There is some variation in opinion as to which musical notes and audio frequencies correspond with each *chakra* – I have included the ones which I have found to be most helpful in my own practice. It's interesting to discuss this with people who facilitate sound healings and gong baths, which can be a wonderful journey into very deep states of relaxation.

Muladhara - **Root Chakra**

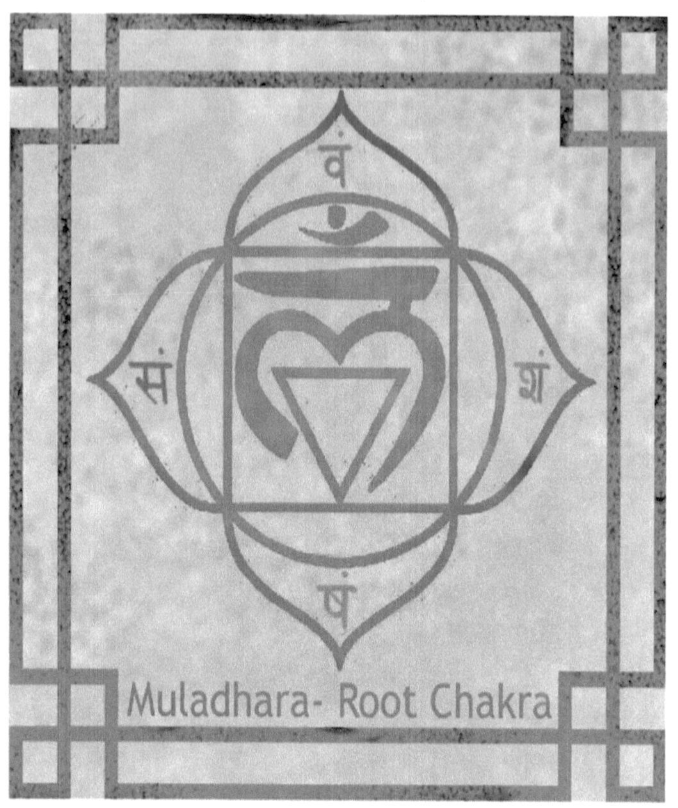

Awareness - survival, safety, basic needs, grounding
When balanced - stability, sense of security, able to trust, self-supporting
In deficiency - fear, anxiety, poor discipline, poor at managing money, eating disorders
In excess - hoarding, lethargy, obesity, constipation, varicose veins
Physical location - perineum
Associated with - skeleton, pelvic floor, legs, feet
Physical function - elimination, balance
Nerve plexus - sacral-coccygeal
Sense - smell
Colour - red
Element - earth
Developmental age - 0-2
Mantra / sound - *Lam*
Frequency / musical note - 108 Hz / A
Mudra - Jnana

Affirmation - I am

Asanas / practices- in deficiency: *Tadasana, Malasana, Uttanasana, Vrksasana, Mula bandha*

- in excess: working with flexibility ie yin yoga; working safely towards postures which are feared ie inversions, backbends, balances

Svastisthana - Sacral Chakra

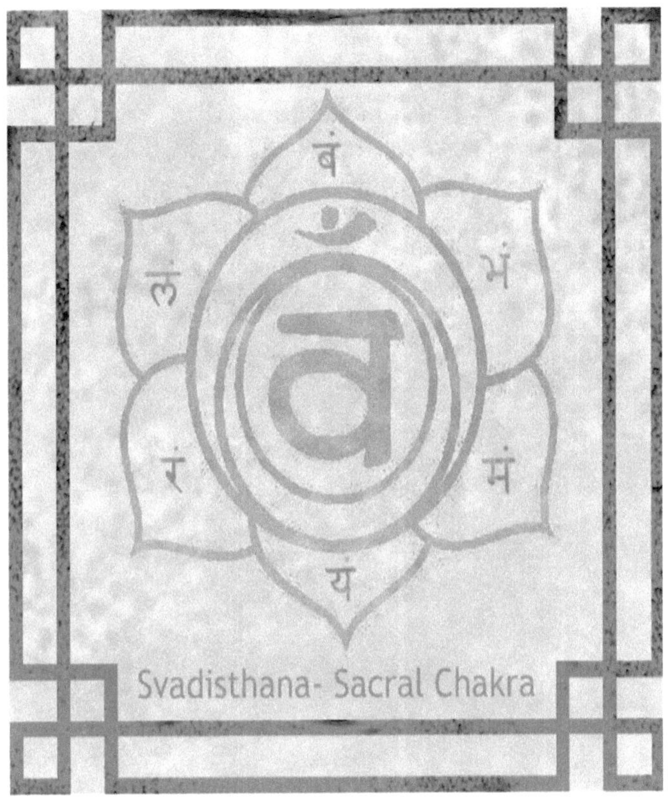

Awareness - self-awareness, sexuality, creativity, self-love

When balanced - creative, comfortable with sexuality / healthy sex life, passion for life

In deficiency - insecurity, oversensitivity, lack of pleasure in life, sexual problems, poor boundaries, menopausal problems

In excess - poor boundaries, creating drama

Physical location - below navel in line with sacrum

Associated with - sacrum, lower back, hips, genitals, womb, bladder, kidneys

Physical function - reproductive system, urogenital, sex hormones

Nerve plexus - sacrolumbar
Sense – taste
Colour - orange
Element - water
Developmental age - 3-7
Mantra / sound - *vam*
Frequency / musical note - 120 Hz / B
Mudra – Yoni
Affirmation - I create
Asanas / practices - in deficiency: *Baddha Konasana, Upavista Konasana, Kati Chalanasana,* being playful/creative - in excess: strengthen *muladhara* and *manipura*; boundary visualisations; creating physical sense of boundaries with use of props ie straps and working with resistance bands.

Manipura - Solar Plexus Chakra

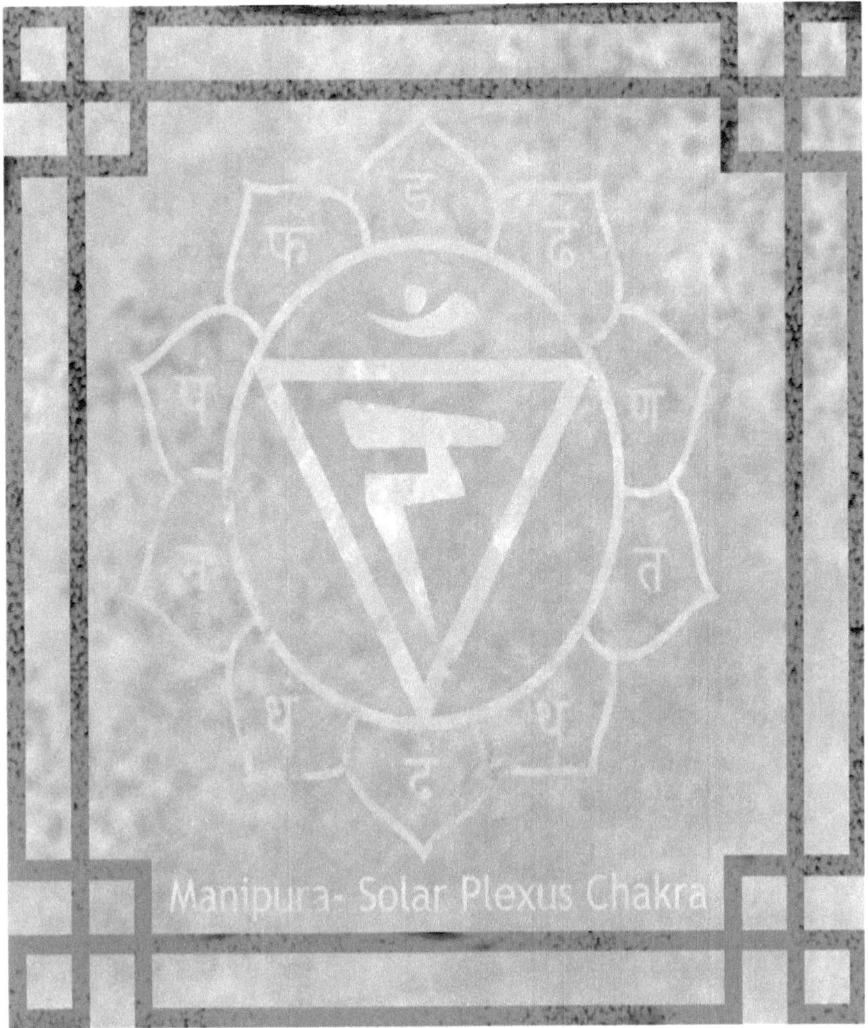

Awareness - courage, willpower, confidence
When balanced - self-confident, self-trusting, takes considered risks, achieves objectives
In deficiency - low self-esteem, lack of self-trust, passivity, chronic fatigue, digestive problems e.g. indigestion
In excess - controlling, competitive, stubborn, aggressive, burns out, over-achieves, digestive problems e.g. acid reflux, ulcers
Physical location - just above navel
Associated with - digestive system, nervous system, skin, adrenal glands

Physical function - assimilation
Nerve plexus - solar plexus
Colour – yellow
Element - fire
Developmental age - 8-18
Mantra / sound – *Ram*
Frequency / musical note - 132 Hz / C
Mudra - Matangi
Affirmation - I will
Asanas / practices- in deficiency: *Surya Namaskar, Virabhadrasana* I and
II, *Uddiyana bandha, Agni Sara, Navasana, Bhastrika pranayama*
- in excess: slowing down and letting go, e.g. restorative postures, yoga nidra,
focus on release of control

Anahata - Heart Chakra

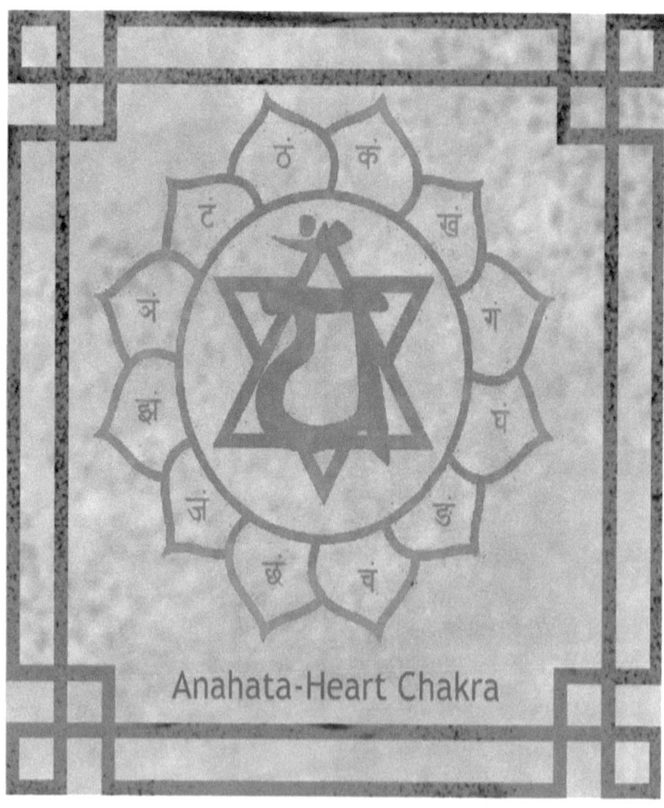

Awareness - love, compassion, forgiveness

When balanced - kind, open to loving and being loved, empathic, compassionate
In deficiency - unkind, lack of compassion, loneliness, jealousy, intolerant, critical, holds grudges, relationship problems, heart and lung disease
In excess - Co-dependency, clinginess, emotionally demanding and high-maintenance
Physical location - behind sternum
Associated with - heart, lungs, chest, upper back, arms, shoulders, thymus gland
Physical function - circulatory and respiratory systems
Nerve plexus - cardiac
Sense – touch
Colour - Emerald green
Element – air
Developmental age - 19-28
Mantra / sound - *Yam*
Frequency / musical note - 150 Hz / D
Mudra - Padma
Affirmation - I love
Asanas / practices - in deficiency: backbends, smiling, positivity, affirmations- in excess: forward bends, self-care, cultivating boundaries and independence
***Vishuddi* - Throat Chakra**

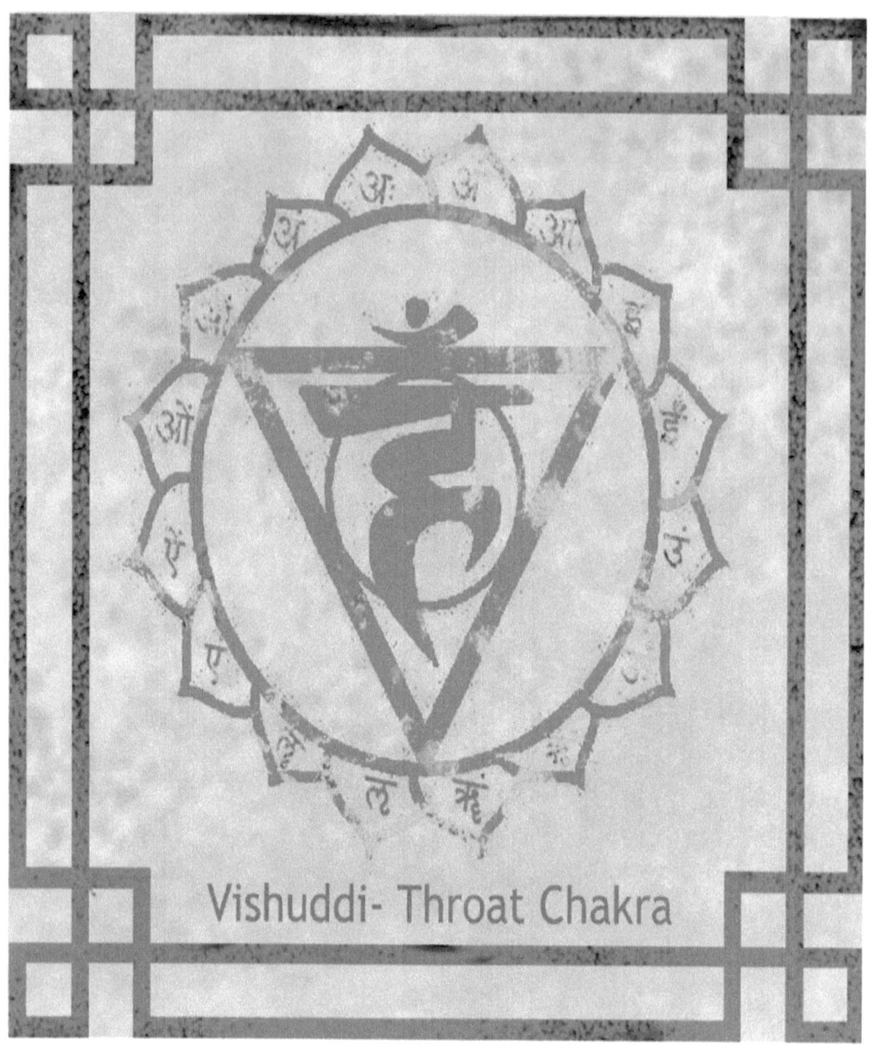

Awareness - communication, self-expression, inspiration
When balanced - strong voice, good listening, in harmony with surroundings
In deficiency - speech problems, throat, neck and mouth problems
In excess - poor listening, excessive talking
Physical location – throat
Associated with - neck, throat, mouth, thyroid and parathyroid glands
Nerve plexus - cervical ganglia medulla
Physical function - respiratory system, speech
Sense – hearing

Colour - turquoise
Element – ether
Developmental age - 29-35
Mantra / sound – *Ham*
Frequency / musical note - 168 Hz / E
Mudra – Shunya
Affirmation - I express
Asanas / practices
- in deficiency: Bridge, Shoulderstand, *Matsyasana*, *Halasana*, *Jalandhara Bandha*, *Ujjayi pranayama*, chanting, Lion's breath
- in excess: spending time in silent meditation or retreat; asking self, before speaking 'Is it true? Is it kind? Is it necessary?'.
***Ajna* - Third Eye Chakra**

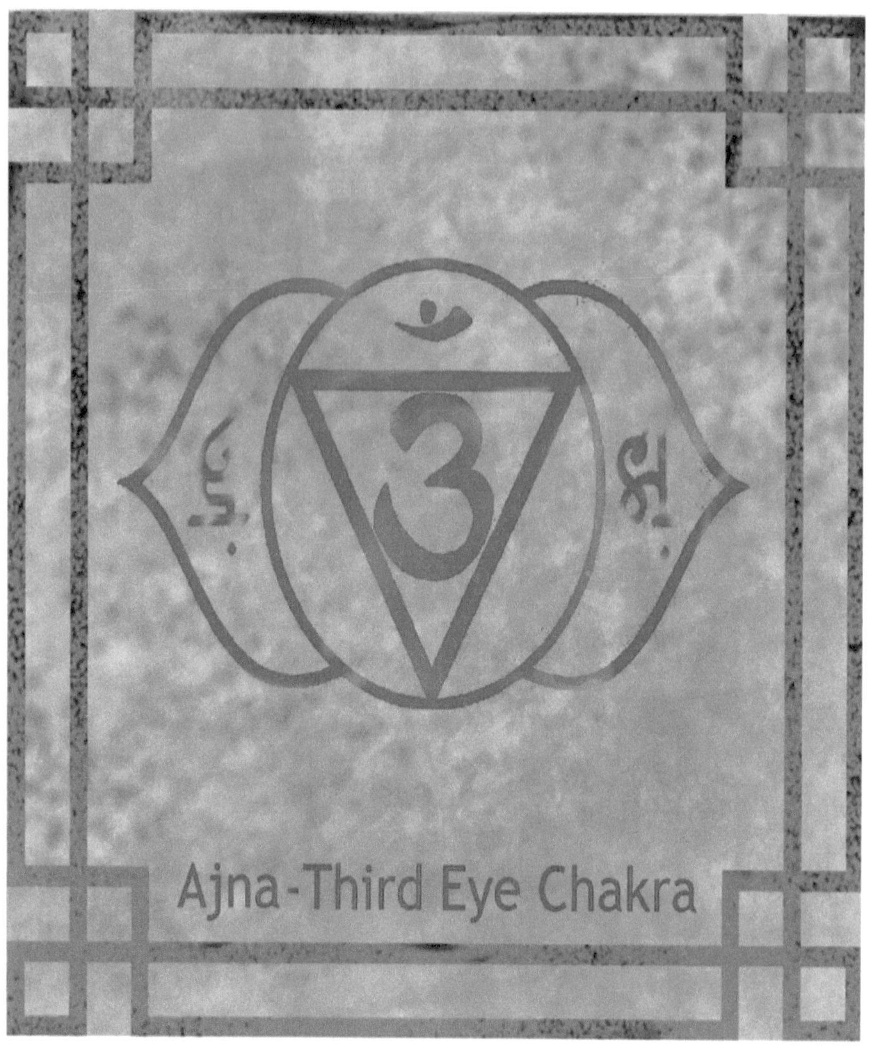

Awareness - intuition, comprehension, insight, perception
When balanced - mental clarity, good intuition
In deficiency - headaches, poor concentration, poor memory, eye problems, poor ability to visualise
In excess - hallucinations, excessive daydreaming, loose grasp on reality
Physical location - between eyebrows, midbrain
Associated with - eyes, pineal gland, central nervous system
Nerve plexus - hypothalamus, pituitary plexus
Physical function - neural messages, sight

Sense - sight
Colour - purple
Element - fire
Developmental age - 36-42
Mantra / sound – *Om*
Frequency / musical note - 180 Hz / F#
Mudra - Dhyana
Affirmation - I see
Asanas / practices
- in deficiency: *Trataka, Balasana, Nadi Shodhana,* visualisation, *Bhramari pranayama,* meditation - in excess: work with lower chakras to balance and ground, e.g. *Hatha* yoga practices; walking barefoot; mindfulness.

Sahasrara - Crown Chakra

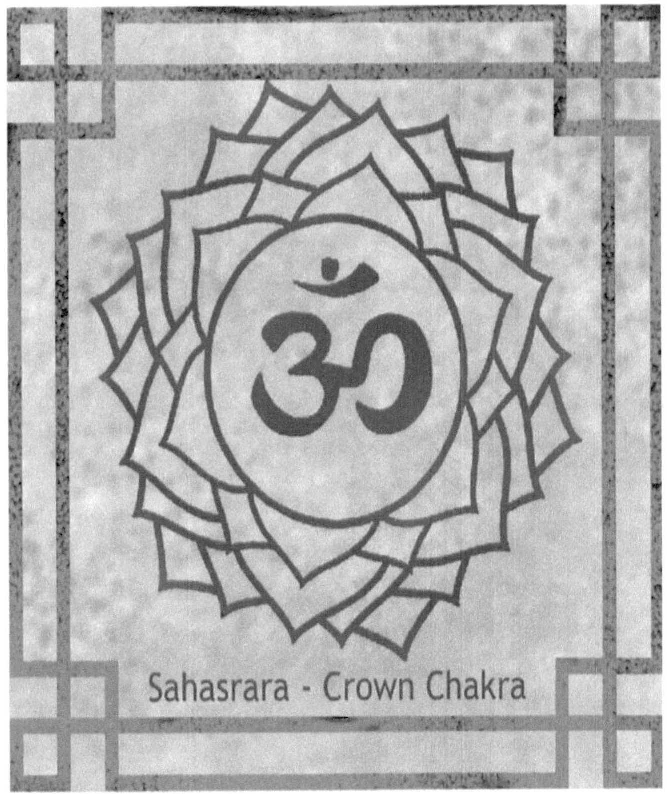

Awareness - spirituality, pure consciousness
When balanced - at peace with self, sense of union with higher power, open

to divine wisdom
In deficiency - materialistic, rejection of spirituality
In excess - spiritual elitism, rigid beliefs
Physical location - crown of head
Associated with - pineal gland
Nerve plexus - cerebral cortex
Sense / sense organ
Developmental age - 43+
Mantra / sound – *Om*
Frequency / musical note - 192 Hz / G
Mudra - Hakini
Affirmation - I connect
Asanas / practices
- in deficiency: Downward Dog, *Sirsasana*, *Padmasana*, chanting *Om*, *Kapalbhati pranayama*, silence, meditation
- in excess: work with lower chakras to balance and ground, e.g. *Hatha* yoga practices; walking barefoot; mindfulness.

But…. are they real?

The *chakras* exist in the subtle energy body, not the anatomical 'meat-suit'. A surgeon can't operate on you and point to your *chakras*. Western society has a somewhat materialistic 'if you can't see it or measure it, it doesn't exist' view of the world – and whilst this may have value in some scientific endeavours, the science of yoga is experiential. If you are having difficulty accepting the concept of *chakras*, I empathise – I was an engineer long before becoming a yogi, and I was decidedly closed-minded to the concept for the first few years of my yoga study. However, after many years of practice and refining my subtle awareness, I embrace the idea simply because I have felt their effects and have first-hand understanding and experience of my own *pranic* body and *chakras*. Being a human is like being a radio with a limited reception bandwidth. Yoga gradually widens this bandwidth so we can perceive what was previously hidden.

Without consciously being aware of it, you have probably felt your own *chakras* at play. Have you ever been so overjoyed or full of love that you could feel it as a physical sensation in the centre of your chest; that your heart felt 'fit to burst'? Have you ever felt a knot of rage in your upper abdomen? How about the fizzing of sexual arousal in the pelvic region? It's an interesting exercise, when you feel a strong emotion, to close your eyes and enquire within as to where you can feel it in your body.

As a start point, you may like to consider the *chakras* as helpful metaphors, or as descriptions of how you conduct yourself and your business in the world. Don't try and make yourself 'believe' in them – simply be open to the idea that there's a great deal in this Universe that we don't understand, go about your practice and they will reveal themselves in time.

The *Prana Vayus*

The movements of energy within us are called the *prana vayus*.

Vayu means wind, so *prana vayus* means energy winds, which refers to the directions of movement of our energy. There are five primary energy motions which encompass the functions of the body's physiological systems, how we feel within ourselves, and how we engage with the world.

Apana vayu

Apana vayu describes a downward and outward motion of energy related to the lower body.

Physically it's to do with elimination of bodily waste, as well as menstruation and childbirth. Psychologically it's associated with releasing what no longer serves us – habits, clutter, old behaviours - and letting go of incidents once they are over rather than carrying baggage. Energetically a healthy *apana vayu* helps us to feel grounded and stable.

An optimally functioning *apana vayu* is of primary importance to the health of the other *vayus* – we have to take out the trash before we concern ourselves with tidying the house!

A weak *apana vayu* might present as (amongst other symptoms) difficulty breathing into the belly; constipation; instability in the lower body; or psychological clinging on to the past / inability to move on.

Practices which stimulate *apana vayu* are diapraghmatic breathing, chanting, strong standing poses such as warriors, forward bends, and child's pose.

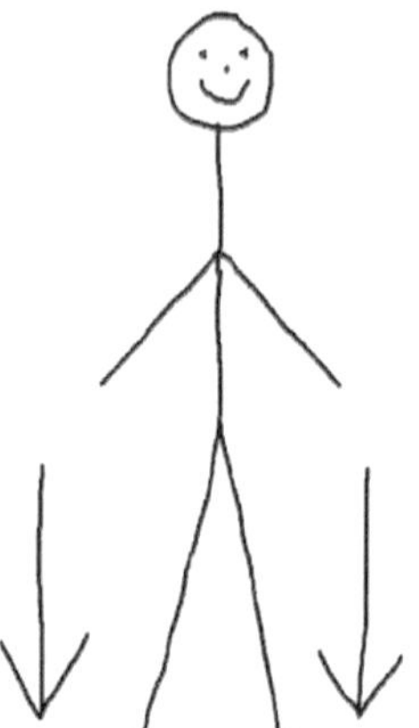

Whilst we refer to all five of the *vayus* collectively as the *prana vayus*, one of them shares the same name in its individual state.

Prana vayu is an inward and upward movement describing the intake of energy, and is related to the body above the diaphragm, ie chest, shoulders, upper back, arms.

We get energy from many different sources such as fresh food, positive relationships, contact with nature, spending time doing things which inspire us and make us feel alive; and of course, breathing. When we have a healthy *prana vayu* we feel energised and vital. If *prana vayu* is lacking, we might feel dull, low in energy, uninspired and lacking in enthusiasm for life.

A weak *prana vayu* might present as chronic fatigue; depression; hunched posture; or upper back problems.

Practices which stimulate *prana vayu* are chest releasing / expanding postures such as side-bends and back-bends, emphasising the inhale, arm movements and all *pranayama*.

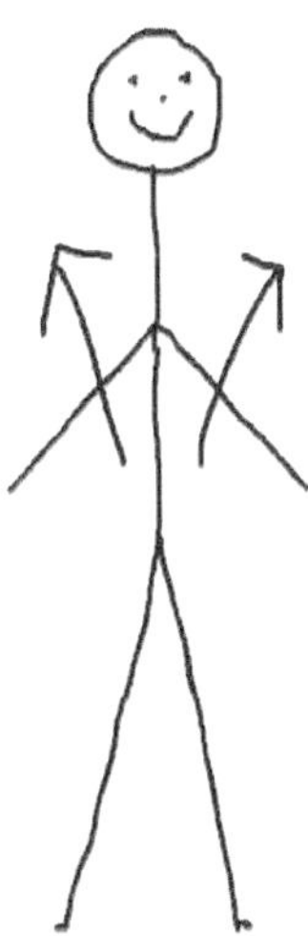

Samana vayu describes a horizontal and centripetal movement of energy, relating to the area between the navel and diaphragm. It is to do with absorption, assimilation, and integration of the energy we take in as well as transformation of all kinds. Physically it has to do with digestion; psychologically and energetically it is associated with balance and discernment – both whether we balance easily on our feet, and whether our lifestyles incorporate appropriate amounts of purposeful work, leisure, rest, learning, creativity, reflection, connection and so on.

A weak *samana vayu* might present as (amongst other symptoms) digestive problems; poor balance; stiffness around the rib cage which restricts the sideways expansion of breathing; poor decision making.

Practices which stimulate *samana vayu* are twists, churning / circular movements, *sama vrtti* (equal fluctuation) breathing, and abdominal work such as *navasana* (boat pose).

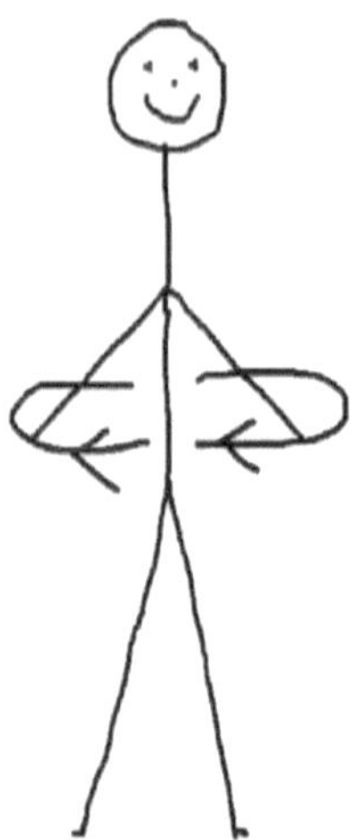

Udana vayu

The upwards and outwards motion of *udana vayu* is the energy of self-expression, enthusiasm and joy, relating to the upper chest, throat, and head. A healthy *udana vayu* helps us to speak expressively and to confidently bring our work and creations into the world, and also to stand tall and feel as though we are 'rebounding' from the Earth's gravitational pull rather than slumping down. Tigger from Winnie the Pooh is the embodiment of *udana* energy!

A weak *udana vayu* might present as (amongst other symptoms) a downcast, shuffling gait or physical 'frozenness'; difficulty in expressing oneself; inability to 'bounce back' from life's challenges; or a weak voice.

Practices which stimulate *udana vayu* are power-posing (standing like Wonder Woman with fists on hips, chest lifted and feet wider than hip distance), inversions, neck movements and *brahmari pranayama* (humming bee breath).

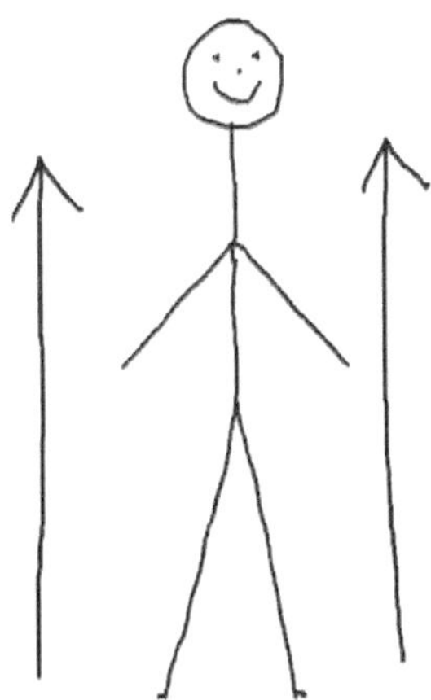

<u>*Vyana vayu*</u>

Vyana vayu is the outwardly circulating energy which moves energy from the centre to the periphery and helps the other *vayus* to move around the whole body. It relates to physical circulation of blood, lymph and nutrients around the body, immunity, and smooth, co-ordinated movements, as well as a sense of steadiness in oneself.

A weak *vyana vayu* might present as (amongst other symptoms) poor circulation; skin problems; poor immunity; or frequent cold feet and hands.

Practices which stimulate *vyana vayu* are flowing whole-body sequences such as sun salutations, rotation of consciousness as in *yoga nidra*, *sharira mudras* and peripheral joint mobilisation (ankles, toes, wrists, fingers).

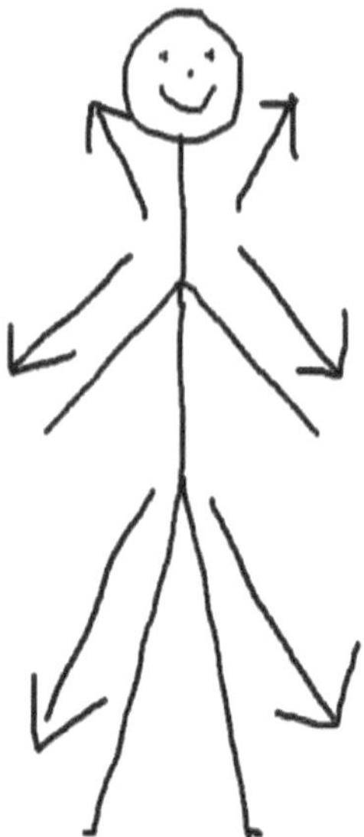

When our energies are nourished and balanced, with ample *prana* in all of the *chakras* and *vayus*, and the *nadis* flowing freely, life feels good. We are calm and full of vitality, able to connect with others and the world around us, and able to bring forth our unique gifts in a way that is meaningful and fulfilling to us. A well-balanced yoga practice comprising all of the limbs, with an emphasis on awareness of our own tendencies and how we feel on a day-to-day, moment-to-moment basis, allows us to come closer to this state of harmony and enjoy life to the full.

The word *guna* means 'strand', and in the yoga tradition the *gunas* form the fabric of existence. They describe the three qualities of nature which make up all matter, energy, and states of mind.

Yoga philosophy relates to but is distinct from the ancient Indian philosophical system called *Samkhya*. The *Samkhya* philosophy states that all which exists can be divided into *prakriti* – matter - and *Purusha* – pure Consciousness. The *gunas* describe the nature of everything that is *prakriti*, including mind.

They are:

Rajas / kriya – vibrancy, motion, dynamism
Tamas / sthiti – dullness, heaviness, inertia
Sattva / prakasha – clarity, luminosity, illumination

These qualities in varying degrees are found throughout all of nature and have their own virtues. They are made manifest in the elements of earth, fire, air, water and space, and in our sense perceptions of smell, sight, touch, taste and sound.

All that exists is subdivided into twenty four *tattvas* or principles in *Samkhya* (other systems such as *Tantra* expand this number). These are:

Prakriti
All of matter, which subdivides into the following:

Three aspects of mind
Ego (*ahamkara)*, intellect (*buddhi*), thinking mind (*manas*)

Five sense organs (*jnanendriyas*)
Nose, eyes, skin, tongue, ears

Five organs of action (*karmendriyas)*
Arms, legs, mouth, reproductive organs, excretory organs

Five senses
Sight, sound, smell, taste, touch

Five gross elements
Earth, fire, air, water, space

The interaction of the *gunas* with the twenty four *tattvas* affects the nature of the manifest world, both animate and inanimate, including the states of the human mind. (*Purusha*, pure Consciousness, is beyond the *gunas*.) This interaction is known as the play of the *gunas*. All three *gunas* are in play at all times, and one will commonly predominate. This is a constantly shifting dance of the natural forces in motion – think of the ongoing changes in daily weather, or fluctuations in our moods. At any time, we might find any one of the *gunas* in dominance over our psychological state. Our thoughts are potential energy, which become habits, desires and consequences of the same nature in the physical world. When the mind's activity is trained and stilled through practice, we can see life more clearly, from a *sattvic* state – we bear witness as the seer. As long as we are identified with our bodies and minds, we are at the mercy of the play of the *gunas*.

Psychological play of the *gunas:*

Tamasic state – inaction, incapacity, ignorance, mechanical routine

Rajasic state – action, passion, effort, struggle, unchanneled power

Sattvic state – equilibrium, harmony, contentment, lucidity

An example of the psychological play of the gunas.

This morning, I was tired and grumpy after a fitful night's sleep full of disturbances. Still, I unwillingly dragged myself out of bed early to go walking and make a call to a friend on the other side of the world as we had agreed, only to receive a message that they couldn't make it. Now I was even grumpier – I could have stayed in bed. As I came back into the house, I narrowly avoided walking on a poop which the cat had thoughtfully left for me inside the door, only to have her squeeze past me and shoot out of the house. This was a problem which roused me to action – we're caring for the cat temporarily and she's not supposed to be outside. I felt panicked as I tried to lure her back in, then chase her, but she was too fast for me and got away. There was nothing I could do but hope she would come home when she got hungry. Still, as my energy levels had suddenly surged, I made use of them and did a dynamic *asana* practice then took a shower. As my mood improved and I was able to see events more clearly, I settled down to do some very enjoyable research, and the cat strolled back in as though nothing had happened. All was right again with my little world and I felt inspired and peaceful.

My morning is an example of how my psychological state shifted from predominantly *tamasic*, to mostly *rajasic,* to largely *sattvic*. Everything that exists, with the exception of *Purusha* (pure Consciousness) is subject to a constantly shifting blend of the *gunas* (whether helpful, agitating, or destructive) from surrounding combinations of forces; and our characters, tempers and reactions are part of this subjectivity.

Sattva is not a balance of *tamas* and *rajas*; rather, it sits above them. *Tamas* is the lowest of the states – according to *Samkhya*, we evolve spiritually from *tamas*, to *rajas*, to *sattva*. However, *sattva* is not the ultimate state – *Purusha* is the eternal witness (Universal Consciousness, soul), and spiritual liberation frees us from the play of the *gunas* entirely, to a state from where Consciousness simply observes as the onlooker, aware but not involved.

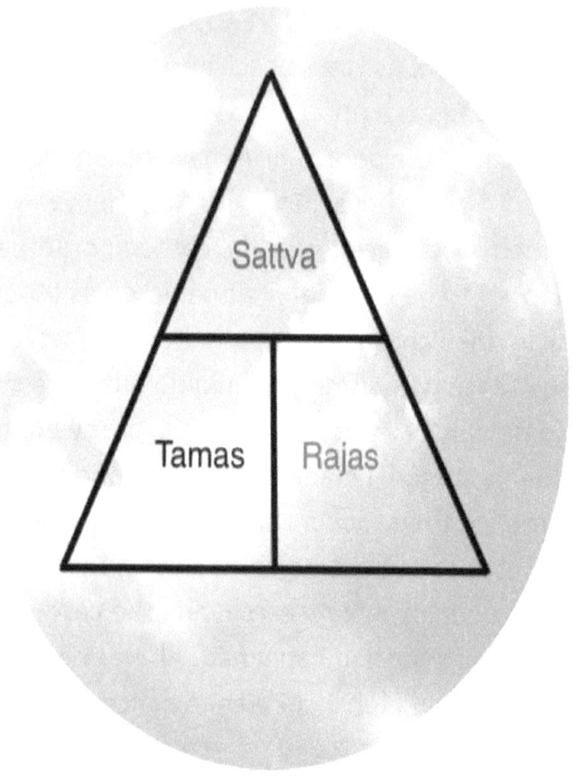

Imagine a glass prism with a beam of light directed on it. Upon contact with the prism the light rays diffract, resulting in the light emerging from the other side in a rainbow of colours spreading out at angles. Now imagine that the original beam of light is the truth of a situation, and the prism is made up of all of your impressions, opinions, misunderstandings, likes and dislikes, life experiences, cultural conditionings, upbringing, fears, and ideas about who you are.

We each see every situation and circumstance through the distortion of our own personal prism, which is unique to us. It's simply impossible for anyone else to see things exactly as you see them because no-one else is you, with the colourations of your experiences, living your life. Recognising this, it's no wonder that there's so much misunderstanding and disharmony in the world!

In sutra 2.2, Patanjali introduces the idea of the *kleshas* (afflictions), as the cause of all human torment and suffering – these are distortions of our own personal prisms. He recommends the practice of yoga as the means to reduce them, and goes on to identify five of these afflictions.

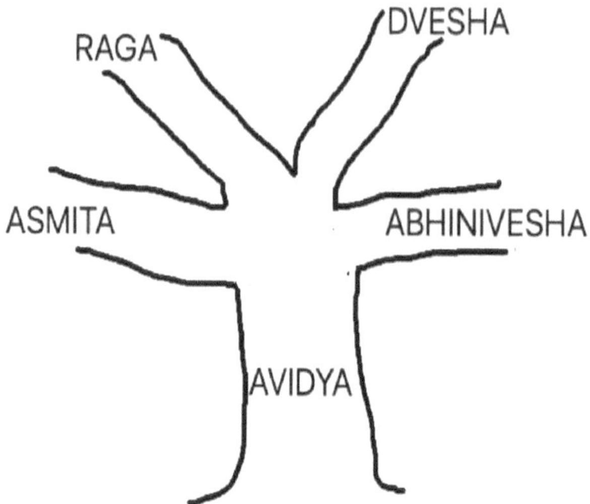

Avidya

If we think of the *kleshas* as a tree, *avidya* is the trunk of the tree and the root of all the other *kleshas*. It means misunderstanding, lack of knowledge, and spiritual ignorance: that is, not knowing who we really are beyond the collection of labels that we stick on ourselves. It is the absence of Self-realisation.

'*Vidya*' means 'truth', in the sense of the ultimate truth of existence as opposed to simple honesty; and the prefix '*a*' in Sanskrit denotes 'not', or 'without'. Therefore '*avidya*' means 'absence of the ultimate truth'. It presents as mistaking the temporary for the permanent, misunderstanding, and misidentification with false identities.

So the first *klesha*, *avidya*, or ignorance of the Self as our true identity, is the primary distortion of how we view the world. Quite simply we misunderstand who we really are, which gives rise to the rest of the *kleshas*.

Asmita

The second *klesha* is *asmita*, or identification with the *ahamkara* ego.

Ego is not just about thinking how wonderful you are and having an over-inflated sense of your own importance. Ego is our identity in the world – it's that description of ourselves as a collection of labels and opinions, our social status, affiliations, education, possessions, roles; it's the view of ourselves as the human being who has impetus and direction in the world. It can be an interesting exercise to view your ego as your human avatar who does their actions in the world and has these values, thoughts, opinions, likes and dislikes. When I know that it's not exactly me, and crucially I know that it's not **all** that I am, I can recognise that I'm a spiritual being having a human experience.

The ego has a major problem in that it functions almost entirely in the past and the future, neither of which actually exist. The only time which ever actually exists is now, the present. You have done things in the past, but when you did them, it was the present. You can make plans to do things in the future, but when the the time comes to actually execute them, it will be the present.

It suits the ego not to recognise this. The ego is exclusively concerned with its own survival, but it has no function when we're in a state of pure Being. It likes to define itself by the collection of things which we have done in the past, by our future plans, because without these, without the labels and definitions, who are we?

We get into trouble when we make the mistake of thinking that we actually *are* the ego-avatar. We suffer huge identity crises when our labels change – if we identify with our job title and think that's who we are, then when we lose that job or retire, we feel like we've lost ourselves and our place in the world. When we define ourselves by the things that we have done, then we live in the past and miss out on the joy of life as it is, right now. If we identify with our mind and believe that our thoughts are truly who we are, then we never know any peace; the mind's activities can be pretty relentless! When we first catch a glimpse of the reality of the situation, and realise that we're actually the one who is watching the thoughts, observing the unfolding of events, it's a quiet revelation. Rather than fighting with our mind and trying unsuccessfully to make it shut up, we can recognise thoughts as passing mental events which have no more substance than a cough or sneeze. We realise that we have a choice about whether or not we engage with the thoughts and fall down the rabbit hole of turning them into a narrative, or whether we allow them to arise and dissolve like bubbles in a glass of soda. We can choose to view our mind as a useful (if rather chatty and opinionated) employee, rather than the big boss! Gradually we develop a sense of ourselves being the awareness behind all of this, and we might find that we can allow each moment to be what it is, without desperately trying to control it. It doesn't mean that we don't take action when action needs to be taken – quite the opposite. In fact, the action that we take from a place of witnessing rather than getting so caught up in personalising random events is of a different quality – wiser, calmer, more compassionate and more effective. When we become aware of our ego-identifications, we find a moment's pause and are more able to sit back in the witness consciousness. We develop the capacity to respond, rather than reacting, and we take action without being attached to our actions having to result in a particular outcome in order for us to be happy.

> Two life-changing books which expand beautifully on this subject are 'The Power of Now' by Eckhart Tolle, and 'The Untethered Soul' by Michael A. Singer.

Patanjali speaks about loosening or weakening our attachments to these ideas of ourselves. It's not that we are trying to totally divest ourselves of human identity, because for us to perform our *dharma* in the world (see chapter 16) we need to be fully functioning human beings with all that that entails. At this level it's a question of finding the balance between recognising ourselves as part of the very fabric of Life itself (and thereby alleviating our mental and existential suffering) and living enjoyable, honourable, human lives in our time here on Earth.

Raga

Raga is all about pleasure; what we like, what we covet and cling to. You've probably heard of 'non-attachment' as being a path to freedom – *raga* is that basis of that attachment.

Of couse, it's normal and natural to have preferences. Even animals have them – a cat might go crazy for a meal of fish but turn her nose up at chicken; a dog will have a favourite toy or place to sleep. That's all perfectly healthy and fine.

The trouble starts when we decide that we can only be happy when those preferences and prejudices are satisfied, and cling to the temporary as if it were permanent – because life will frequently not co-operate with granting our desires, and everything changes, all the time. In yoga philosophy, the only permanent thing is Consciouness itself. Everything else is subject to change – indeed, change is the only constant. So when we try and deny this to ourselves; when we want each pleasurable experience to last forever, when we try to hold onto people, circumstances, even our own bodies as they age, then we inevitably suffer. Through the practices of yoga, particularly the study of philosophy, of our own psychology (*svadhyaya*), and regular meditation, we gradually become aware of where we cling and we become more accepting of the transience of all things. There is nothing wrong with enjoying life's pleasures – life is a journey to be enjoyed! But learning to hold the things we like lightly, and enjoy them wholeheartedly in the full knowledge that they are impermanent, is a path to greater mental freedom and happiness.

<u>What the Sutras Say</u>

Sutra 1.15 *Drsta anusravika visaya vitrsnasya vasikarasamjna vairagyam*

This sutra tells us that 'at the highest level of consciousness, there is freedom from craving and desires'.

<u>Dvesha</u>

The fourth klesha, *dvesha*, is the flip-side of *raga*. *Dvesha* is aversion, revulsion, dislike; anything we keenly want to avoid. When we're entangled in *dvesha*, we become intolerant of any person and situation not meeting our expectations. We require everything to be 'just so', and the slightest deviation from everything being exactly the way we want it throws us off course. As life is rarely so favourably disposed, we set ourselves up for a world of hurt!

Strong aversions can arise as the result of an association of particular situations and objects with painful past experiences. There might no longer be any reason for the aversion once circumstances have changed, yet still they persist. Can we observe our own tendencies to mentally slam the door on certain things when there is no longer any reason to do so, and so reassess our behaviour, particularly if it limits us? For example, perhaps as a child you trod on a sea urchin and so have avoided swimming in the ocean ever since. Is that association and aversion still limiting your experience many years later? Perhaps you have been hurt in a romantic relationship, and so rather than risk being vulnerable again, you avoid getting close to people and suffer a feeling of loneliness as a result. Does one unkind partner mean that all potential partners are unkind, or does an aversion that causes you suffering warrant a little investigation?

Like its predecessor, *raga*, there's no problem with having preferences and mild aversions, as long as we don't become ruled by them. Personally I really dislike the taste of parsley, but if I order a dish in a restaurant and it comes sprinkled with the stuff, I can just scrape it off – no need to get upset. If someone cuts me off in traffic I might feel angry right then, but there's no need to carry the annoyance around with me and let it ruin my day after the moment has passed.

A yoga practice helps us to feel that we have inside of us an ever-present refuge of peace. We recognise that most unfavourable circumstances really don't matter and need not disturb us, and that events are simply what they are – it's only our own mental constructs that label them good or bad.

> 'There is nothing either good or bad,
> but thinking makes it so.'
> Hamlet – William Shakespeare

Both aversion and attachment require the overactive sense of 'I – ness' of ego-identification in order to exist; which in turn requires that we are caught in the confusion and misunderstanding of ignorance.

<u>Abhinivesha</u>

The final *klesha, abhinivesha,* is insecurity and fear – especially our primal fear of death (both our own and others). Most animals, humans included, strongly dislike insecurity and uncertainty - and yet this is the very nature of life. Everything is impermanent.

As life progresses, a sustained yoga practice helps us to sense that we are a part of the universal energy that surounds us; that whilst our bodies change and eventually deteriorate, life and death are two sides of the same coin, and that it is death which ultimately gives life its meaning. Yoga - meaning 'unity' - invites us to experience a sense that this energy which is 'me', this spark of Consciousness which is the Self, is like a drop of water temporarily distinguished from the ocean as a raindrop. Upon falling back into the ocean we see that it's not really separate at all. Death is a great uniter – we all lose loved ones, we will all die ourselves. Do we really have to fear death? Or would it be wiser to wake up and live fully - to fear not dying itself, but dying without ever having woken up and truly lived?

Again, in order for this fear to have us in its grip, we need to be ignorant of our true Self, and over-identified with ego.

I am unaware that my true nature is Life itself (*avidya*)

So I attach to an ego identity (*asmita*)

Which tries to cling to favourable things (*raga*)

And avoid unfavourable things (*dvesha*)

And is fundamentally insecure so lives in fear (*abhinivesha*)

Every one of us has our own special brew of these five *kleshas:* our misapprehension, ego-identity, attachments, aversions and fears, which develop through our unique set of life experiences, circumstances, and the family and wider culture in which we're raised. We each experience the world through this prism, and no two people will ever see everything in the same way. A regular yoga practice can help us to become familiar with the constitution of our own prism and catch glimpses of seeing clearly. Gradually we develop an awareness of our own blind-spots. We realise that everyone else has their own story, which is just as much a part of their experience as ours is to us, and that helps us to develop a sense of compassion, acceptance and equanimity towards ourselves and others.

We are unlikely to ever rid ourselves of the *kleshas*, and even Patanjali talks of diminishing and weakening them ahead of fully divesting ourselves of them. They are an evolutionary imperative which developed for a reason – a sense of ourselves as individual personalities with unique attributes helps us to fulfil our *dharma* or purpose in the world (see chapter 16); likes and dislikes can steer us towards sensible *viveka* or wise discernment so as to use what is helpful and steer clear of what is damaging; and without fear of insecurity and death we wouldn't have evolved very far at all because we'd take foolish risks and get ourselves killed. The key is to become more self-aware and recognise when a particular *klesha* is over-active and causing us suffering. Recognising our own tendencies and shortcomings is a vital part of our spiritual evolution into a more liberated way of life, with far less self-created suffering.

Chapter 15 – Psychology of Yoga: The Obstacles to Yoga

In Sutra (1.30), Patanjali describes the nine principle obstacles which stand between us and living in the state of peace and clarity which is yoga. These obstacles are often manifestations of suffering brought about by the *kleshas*.

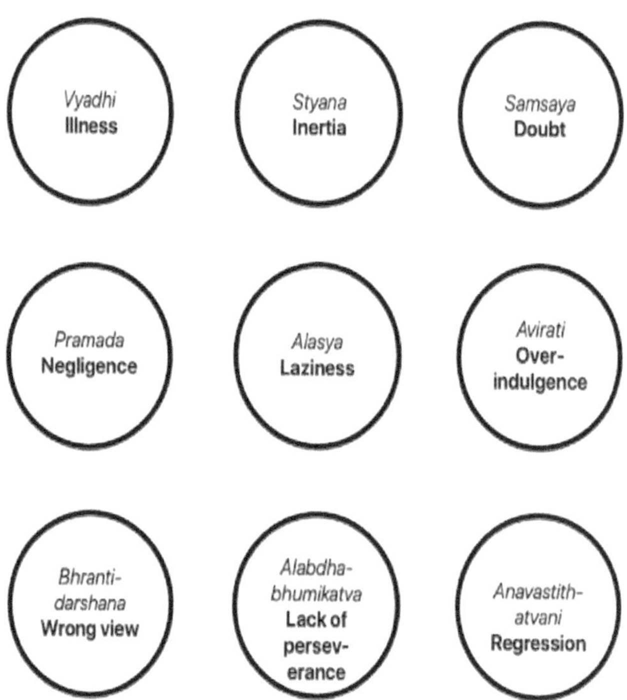

The obstacles are:

Vyadhi – sickness

When we're unwell, our physical state of feeling weak and sick is a clear impediment to finding steadiness of mind – we're distracted by our pain and discomfort and our energy levels are low or erratic.

Styana - inertia, lack of motivation, rigidity

Feeling lethargic and apathetic – which may arise from ill-health – is an obvious obstacle. We need a little get-up-and-go to engage with life and our yoga practice or we procrastinate; and rigidity of mind means that we struggle to adapt to new situations or believe that we have the capacity to change and grow of our own volition.

Samsaya – **doubt, uncertainty**

Many of us have experienced imposter syndrome - an unpleasant voice in our heads which says we're not good enough and that we should just give up. Equally we might lose faith in the value of practice and think that what we're doing is pointless.

Pramada – **negligence, rushing, carelessness**

'Slow and steady wins the race'. Slowing down, paying attention and undertaking tasks with care, precision and concentration means fewer mistakes and better quality of actions.

Alasya – **laziness**

Sloth and lack of willpower obstruct the way every time when we can't be bothered to do what we know is best for us.

Avirati – **overindulgence**

Succumbing to the lure of sense-attachments is a particular jeopardy in the Western world where we are constantly encouraged by advertising to eat this, drink that, buy the other. Such 'luxuries' are no such thing though, if they adversely affect our wellbeing - for example by making us feel sluggish, or result in financial anxiety because we're living beyong our means.

Brantidarshana - **wrong view; illusion**

After a few years of practice we may fall into the trap of thinking we know it all. Many years later we may realise how little we truly grasp. 'The phrase 'I don't know' is the beginning of wisdom.

Alabdhabhumikatva – **lack of perseverance**

Yoga requires steady, sustained and enthusiastic practice over time. 'Little and often' yields far richer progress than inconsistent and sporadic attempts.

Anavasithatvani - **regression into old ways**

Changes in lifestyle choices tend to arise naturally on the path of yoga, but it's easy to get tempted back into old habits which impede our progress. The important thing is to treat ourselves with friendliness when we fall off the horse, and simply get back on without retribution.

All of these obstacles, which tend to be brought about by the existence of strong *kleshas*, are as relevant to life today as they were when the Sutras were committed to text. Patanjali goes on to explain that the four symptoms of the presence of any one of these obstacles are pain/suffering; despair; unsteadiness of the body; and irregular breathing.

What the Sutras Say

Sutra 1.29 *Tatah pratyakcetana adhigamah api anatarya abhavah ca*

Meditation on *Om* removes obstacles to the mastery of the inner self.

We may also work towards overcoming these obstacles and symptoms by weakening the *kleshas*, through keen effort in practice.

Samskaras* and *Vikalpas

In addition to these obstacles and the *kleshas*, there are two more psychological plights which can impede our ability to see clearly, called *samskaras* and *vikalpas*.

A *samskara* is an impression. From early childhood we receive and form impressions about ourselves and the world around us, and when we repeatedly receive an impression it makes a slightly deeper impact every time. Think about a car driving over wet grass. The first time, the grass will be flattened and you'll be able to see light tyre tracks where the car has been. After driving over the same spot a few more times, the grass will start to get squashed down into the earth and definite tracks will be visible. If the car keeps going over the same spot, deep grooves are made in the mud which will eventually become trenches. This is how our minds behave when we repeatedly receive an impression – neural pathways are formed and strengthened and the impression becomes deep and abiding. This can be useful, for example when using repetition to learn something (like how to drive a car). But impressions are not limited to learning new skills; they include ideas and judgements, and result in a rigid way of thinking and perceiving the world, where we are unreceptive and closed-minded to contradictory ways of seeing things. Eventually, if samskaras are not challenged, we can become 'set in our ways'; stale and inflexible of mind.

Samskaras are closely related to *vikalpas*, which are mental constructs. Like *samskaras*, *vikalpas* are a necessary part of being human – they give us the ability to imagine and plan. For example, because I have a mental construct of where I need to go to, I can plan my journey. However they have a downside, which is that our ability to imagine can result in us making up stories and acquiring erroneous, false, and limiting beliefs about ourselves and the world around us. Perhaps as a child you were repeatedly told to keep your voice down and were punished for being rambunctious; that may form a limiting belief in your subconscious that you'll get in trouble if you behave enthusiastically or speak up for yourself, and mean that you spend your life being limited by timidity. Someone may make an unkind remark about your body that stays with you and becomes a 'fact' in your head, when in reality it's no such thing. Everyone has beliefs like this, some of which may be damaging and some which may be helpful. The same belief can even be either helpful OR harmful depending on who holds it – a belief that 'hard work reaps dividends' might amply serve someone who is working on a craft that they love; or equally keep someone banging their head against a wall in a job they hate. Once formed it may be impossible to totally eliminate a *vikalpa*, but what we can do is discover which of these 'background programs' are running in the computers of our minds, and challenge the validity of any that are holding us back from realising our true purpose and potential. Once we know what's in our subconscious, we are far less likely to be caught out by it. Then we can find a sankalpa which writes a more helpful program to live by, and by working consciously to strengthen that, dramatically improve the quality of our own inner lives.

Chapter 16 – Psychology of Yoga: *Dharma* and the *Purusharthas* - True purpose and our human aims

Is there anything more fulfilling than living your true purpose?

If Yoga as a whole is about Self-**realisation** (capital S), which is a spiritual awakening to the sense of our higher selves as part of a much greater whole, then individual *dharma* could be said to concern self-**actualisation** (small s) – the bringing forth of our unique human talents and aptitudes for the good of all beings.

It has been said that yoga is a journey of the self (small s), through the self (small s), to the Self (large S). We develop our ability to act skilfully in the world for the highest good of all beings, alongside deepening our awareness of ourselves as something more than simply our human forms.

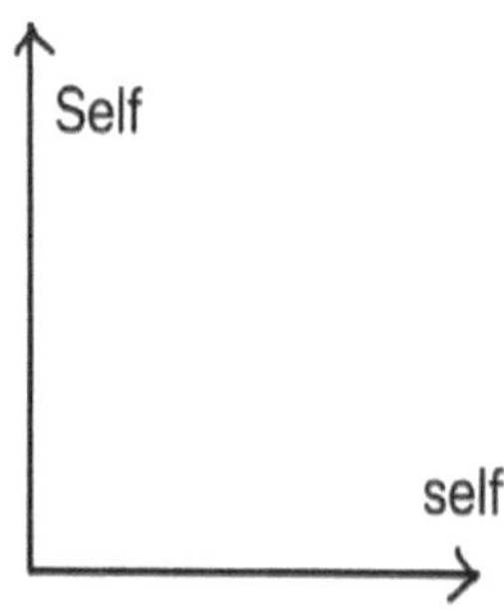

Dharma is a concept found in Yoga (in the Vedas), Buddhism and Hinduism, and it describes a principle which governs and sustains the Universe – the organising principle of the cosmos. The planets circle the sun, rain falls to Earth, children become adults, fish swim, birds fly, fire is hot – you get the idea. Like everything else, we humans have our roles to play. We are each a tiny slice of the Universe experiencing itself through our current form, and the understanding of our individual *dharma* answers that most fundamental of human enquiries: 'why am I here?' Living in accordance with the principle of *dharma* means using our abilities to serve humanity and help others.

When we as individuals live our *dharma*, we live in alignment with this principle of life's intrinsic inner wisdom, following our true calling and serving all other beings by playing our unique role. The idea is that we each have a special purpose in our time here – a duty to ourselves, the people around us, and the wider world - and that we come equipped with the necessary attributes to fulfil this purpose. Individual *dharma* is our soul's calling. To live without realising your *dharma* is to feel deep down that you're living someone else's life; that on some level you're not being true to your purpose. Supporting our individual *dharma* means living a life which is in harmony with the larger cosmic principle .

'Why are you acting so small? You are

the Universe in ecstatic motion.'

Rumi

There are many ways to express our *dharma*, and the way in which we uphold it will be determined by our values and the things we enjoy doing. For example, a person's *dharma* may be to gather and share knowledge; there are many different ways in which they could do this. They might become a primary school teacher, research scientist, university lecturer, non-fiction writer, orator, TV documentary presenter, business advisor, and so on. Equally they may choose a job which doesn't at first glance fulfil their *dharma*, but find a way to shift the way in which they work to encompass it – for example, by mentoring less experienced colleagues or setting up training programs. Alternatively they might express it in their free time, perhaps by volunteer teaching in developing countries during their holidays if they loved to travel, or starting a local allotment group if gardening and self-sufficiency held a keen interest for them. *Dharma* **may** involve career as that is where we spend a lot of our time, but it does not **necessarily** have to do so. There are many ways of aligning our purpose with an existing role, and it may be a question of simply changing the **way** we do something, rather than changing the thing itself.

Personally it took me over forty years to understand my *dharma*, even though I was already living it without realising, as many of us will. Mine is to serve others by helping them to feel comfort and ease in their environments. There are countless ways in which I could express this! Professionally, I work as a yoga therapist and coach which means I help people to find comfort and ease in all aspects of their being – both throughout their *koshas*, which we explored in chapter 1 – and in their wider lives. I run yoga reatreats, which are all about creating an environment for people to connect with themselves on a deeper level and feel deeply relaxed and rejuvenated. I also work as a sound engineer, mixing monitor sound for live bands, which means that I am responsible for what the band hear on stage. I make sure that the musicians can hear a high quality mix of themselves and each other so that they can relax and do their job of giving a great performance. These are the methods which appeal to me, but I was able to fulfil it through my job when I worked in a pub (by cheerfully chatting with and crucially, **listening to** customers), and I could find ways to express it in virtually any workplace simply by the **way** I do the job, and the attitude and quality of attention I bring to it. It's also not just about work! I can fulfil my *dharma* of helping others feel at ease when I'm not working too – I can smile at passers-by, chat to the new person in a yoga class to help them feel included, give a home to rescue animals, create a peaceful living environment for my family, and so on.

The method we choose to express our *dharma* is informed by our interests, values and talents. The way you express your *dharma* is as unique as your fingerprint. What's more, you can't always tell from the outside if someone is living theirs (unless they're totally miserable for years on end – that's a pretty good sign that they're not).

Let's say you've worked as a retail manager for many years. You're good at the job and well-respected, but it doesn't inspire you and you have a nagging feeling of 'is this it?' You do it for the paycheque but you just can't wait for the weekends when you can pack up your camping gear and go hiking in the hills, where you spend hours absorbed in sketching the views and your soul feels alive. A process of self-enquiry leads you to realise that your *dharma* is to share the life-enhancing, health-regenerating beauty of the great outdoors.

One option to fulfil your dharma could be to train as a mountain leader and take groups on hiking expeditions. Another could be to sell your sketches. However, if you have a family to support, that may not bring in enough money to be practical – *dharma* is also about duty and meeting our responsibilities. But perhaps you could research hiking and outdoor stores who are looking for a manager – your passion for the subject would shine through and you could advise customers on the best equipment, routes, and safety skills. Perhaps you could create postcards from your sketches and sell them in store, give occasional workshop-style talks, or even spend some of your weekends training to lead expeditions so that you're fully qualified when the kids are grown. That's a route that would surely leave you feeling vastly more fulfilled and aligned with your purpose, all whilst taking care of those around you.

According to the yoga tradition, we have four types of desire called the *purusharthas*. They are *dharma, artha, kama,* and *moksha.*

Dharma is our soul's purpose, our reason for being in the world, our duties here on Earth. By being true to it we bring forth the unique nugget hidden within us, the unique expression of the Universe that we are.

Artha is the desire to bring about the means to enable us to answer our soul's calling and fulfil our practical needs and responsibilities such as keeping a roof over our family's head, keeping ourselves and our environment clean, doing our work to bring in an income to live and therefore birth our expression in the world. Artha encompasses the pursuit of our chosen profession or vocation.

Kama is the desire for pleasure, love, and the cultivation of artistic and cultural pursuits. There's no problem with pleasure as long as we don't become attached to having it. There's nothing wrong with liking good food, or music, or art, or sex, or beautiful surroundings, so long as we can hold them lightly – the world and all its wonders are here to be connected with and enjoyed.

Moksha is the desire for liberation, the yearning for spiritual freedom which leads us down this path of exploration and self-discovery.

These four needs are part and parcel of the human journey, and whilst one of them is usually predominant depending on our stage of life, optimal satisfaction and contentment arises as a balance of all four, preferably with a taste of each of them in every day. *Dharma* is the main desire, which could be said to give rise to the others. *Dharma* and *moksha* are the two which are most directly addressed by yoga practices, but a balance between all of them is the key to a happy and fulfilling life.

The famous text of the *Bhagavad Gita* is a story which centres around the idea of *dharma*. It takes place on a battlefield, as a conversation between a young prince, Arjuna, and his charioteer who is actually Lord Krishna. Krishna advises Arjuna that it is better to do one's own *dharma* poorly, than to do another's well.

If you wake up looking forward to the day's tasks and have a feeling of being aligned with how you spend your time; if your life feels fulfilling and there is no sense of having missed your calling or longing to be elsewhere; then chances are you are already living your purpose or pretty close to it.

The trick to finding your purpose is to keep following the clues. You have to wake up enough to start noticing the moments when you feel most alive, and ask them what they're trying to tell you. You have to 'follow the strange pull of what you really love; it will not lead you astray'.

That's where the mind-steadying and self-enquiry parts of yoga come in. Intuition is a voice without words – a 'gut feeling' – and it's very hard to access it when we're stuck in our own heads. Yoga gives us a time-out from that, a way to find some space to listen to our inner wise person. Self-enquiry – the third *niyama* of *svadhyaya* – is an opportunity to ask ourselves the kind of searching questions which we may never explore in normal western living, and so connect with our life's true purpose as a tiny part of the fabric of the Universe – our *dharma*.

Three steps towards finding your *dharma*

1 – Start noticing the moments when you feel excited, as though you're lit up from the inside. What are you doing at those times, when you feel so joyous? Can you bring more of those things into your life? The clues to your *dharma* lie in the things that make you feel genuinely enthusiastic and most alive.

2 – Start to also pay attention to moments when you feel the opposite! I don't mean the things that you just find a bit dull but which are necessary, like (for example) doing housework, but the moments when you feel deflated, drained of vitality, or as though a tiny bit of you just died. Is it time to say 'no' to some of these things, to make space in your life for the things that make you come alive?

3 – Start noticing the little coincidences and things that seem to regularly pop up in your life unprompted. When you start to align with your purpose, life has a funny way of oiling the wheels.

No-one else can tell you what your *dharma* is (although they may well try!). But as huge and daunting as discovering your life's purpose may sound, finding your *dharma* need not be a terrifying proposition and can actually be an enormously enjoyable project of *svadhyaya* (self- enquiry). The process of discovery was encapsulated by 13th century poet Rumi when he said:

**'Follow the strange pull of what you really
love; it will not lead you astray.'**

For further reading and self-enquiry practices on this subject you may like 'The Four Desires' by renowned teacher Rod Stryker.

Chapter 17 – Your Yoga Journey - incorporating these concepts into your own practice and life

We've met a great many concepts throughout this book, but they're only of use if they help us in our day-to-day lives. Remember, the purpose of yoga is to alleviate suffering and lead us towards Self-realisation. So how can we use each of these yogic tools and philosophies to enhance our modern lives?

Let's briefly recap our journey together from the top, and see how we can apply some of the things we've explored.

<u>The *Koshas* (Chapter 1)</u>

We began with the idea of ourselves as multi-dimensional beings, which is fundamental to understanding why and how yoga works. A great way to regularly check in with these aspects of yourself is to contemplate these questions:

- How does my body feel, and what could I do to help that part of me?
- How does my energy and life-force feel, and what could I do to help that part of me?
- How does my mind feel, and what could I do to help that part of me?
- How am I experiencing the wisest part of myself, and what could I do to connect with that?
- How am I experiencing the part of me that is pure Presence and joy, beyond time and space, and what could I do to connect with that?

<u>The *Yamas* and *Niyamas* (Chapters 3 and 4)</u>

The five *yamas* (universal observances) and five *niyamas* (personal observances) are our guidelines for ethical living.

The *yamas* are:

Ahimsa – non-violence
Satya – truthfulness
Asteya – non-stealing
Brahmacharya – continence

Aparigraha – non-grasping / letting go

The *niyamas* are:

Saucha – cleanliness / purity
Santosha – contentment
Tapas – burning enthusiasm / discipline
Svadhyaya – self-enquiry
Ishvara Pranidhana – surrender to a greater force

In chapters 2 and 3 you'll find plenty of practical suggestions for putting each of these principles into practice in modern life. A really effective way to help them 'take root and bear fruit' in your life is to focus on each principle in turn for a week at a time, and contemplate where in your own life you can more effectively honour it. This is how we begin to bring yoga into every aspect of our lives – we can live yoga all day long, not just when we're on the mat!

<u>Asana – Chapter 5</u>

If you take regular yoga classes then *asana* – postures – is probably an aspect of yoga which features prominently in your life. Make sure that your practice stays true to yoga and doesn't become mere gymnastics by enquiring into the following:

- Do you find *sthira* (steadiness) and *sukha* (ease) throughout your practice, even in the transitions between poses?

- Is your breath *dirgha* (long) and *sukshma* (smooth)?

- Is your breath leading the movement (breath begins, movement follows; movement ends, then breath ends) or has the relationship between breath and movement become mechanical?

- Is your mind focused on this breath, this body, this movement?

It's also good to make sure your practice is balanced by ensuring that it moves your spine in all four directions (forward, back, side to side, twist).

Asana helps us to cultivate a healthy, comfortable, relaxed body; an enjoyable place to live as spiritual beings having a human experience.

<u>Pranayama – Chapter 6</u>

Pranayama – breathwork, or literally 'extension of the life-force' – is a vital component of yoga. Our breath is the bridge between body, energy, and mind; its quality and behaviour hold important clues to our wellbeing, and our ability to shape it is the key to better health and a quieter mind. The more times you check in with how you're breathing and take a moment to make the flow slower and fuller, the better. A good way to incorporate this is to choose something that happens multiple times throughout your day, such as standing up from your desk, checking your phone, or making a drink, and get into the habit of observing your breath just for a few moments. Then take three really slow, full breaths before continuing about your business. By creating this tiny habit, you'll become generally more aware of how you're breathing, and be reminded to breathe more fully. Having the ability to profoundly alter your own nervous system – like switching yourself from fight and flight into the relaxation response in stressful situations – is one of the simplest and most valuable tools that yoga has to offer us. As your practice advances you may discover a particular *pranayama* technique which becomes your 'go-to' – I often find myself using *Ujjayi pranayama* when I'm in high-pressure situations, and it makes me feel instantly calmer and more grounded.

> Remember: If you **mimic** a relaxed and happy state with your body, face and breathing, your brain and nervous system have no choice but to follow suit.

Pratyahara – Chapter 7

True *pratyahara* – withdrawal from the senses – tends to be a state which arises as a result of practice and/or intense concentration rather than something you just 'do'. However, in a more prosaic sense there are simple ways in which we can reduce the impact of our senses on our inner world. Personally I like to use foam earplugs when I'm travelling on trains or planes to give me some respite from external noise (note that this is not the same as listening to headphones, because then you are still listening). Using an eye pillow during your *savasana* as the end of *asana* practice is also a pleasant touch of sense-withdrawal in our busy days, allowing us to more readily access our 'inner retreat'. And simply shifting our perspective to realise that we are in control of what we give our attention to, and that we can choose to focus on one thing and ignore another, is a crude form of pratyahara.

<u>Dharana</u> – Chapter 8

Dharana is concentration, and learning to concentrate is nothing more than practice. There's no fancy mystery to it, you just have to decide to focus on something, and then every time you realise your mind has wandered off, bring it back without remonstrating with it! Of course, the combination of *asana* and breath, with additions such as *drishti* (gaze point) or visualisation, serve to keep the mind occupied and attentive to the task at hand. But we can practice improving our concentration skills all day long, we don't have to be on the yoga mat.

If concentrating is a struggle for you, it can be helpful to first write down a to-do list of all the things you're likely to remember when you're trying to concentrate. This is a really great thing to do in the morning to help you stay focused all day. Your mind is just trying to help, and writing things down lets it relax.

As a general rule for improving concentration, the more multi-dimensional the thing you have to concentrate on, the easier it is. (Note that this is NOT the same thing as multi-tasking, which usually results in us doing multiple things badly rather than one thing well!) Single activities which require the co-ordination of different skills or faculties such as sketching, playing an instrument, learning a language, playing tennis, reading aloud, knitting, or learning a dance routine engage your 'executive function' pre-frontal cortex rather than something you can easily zone out to like walking or listening to a podcast. Start with committing to pay attention for very small periods of time - 5 minutes perhaps - then build it up as your concentration muscle gets stronger and you become more accomplished at gathering all your mental energy and directing it to a particular task.

This is how you train your mind to become your helpful servant rather than feeling like you're hitched to a runaway train! This is a powerful step to vastly better mental wellbeing, and a key to the door of that longed-for jewel of yoga - inner peace.

<u>Dhyana</u> – Chapter 9

Like *pratyahara*, true *dhyana* – meditation – is a state that arises rather than something you can just sit down and 'do'. Most commonly when we 'meditate' we're actually practising concentrating, which steadies the mind and gradually leads it into an increasingly quiet and unfluctuating state. I cannot recommend highly enough forming a daily meditation practice. I'm in my tenth year of meditating first thing every morning, and I find it a wonderful way to start the day which has dramatically improved my life. I sit for 30-40 minutes now, but I began with just ten conscious breaths each day. Start small, keep it simple, and follow the golden 'new habit' rule of linking it with an existing part of your routine, and you'll soon find that it becomes a valuable part of your life which keeps you closely connected to your practice.

<u>*Samadhi* – Chapter 10</u>

Samadhi – merging into bliss – is the ultimate state of yoga; a complete sense of union with life and immersion into the Universe. It's certainly a lofty aim, but it's important to remember that a yoga journey is not linear. It ebbs and flows; some days it's easier to feel close to touching that state and on others it feels a million miles away. The truth is that it is always here; it's our natural underlying state before we heap all of our human troubles and neuroses upon it and so lose sight of it. Try to make time every day to do the things or be in the places where you most readily find a sense of peace and ease. For many of us that means being in nature, and if you live in a city you can still take a moment to sit back and look up at the sky. You might find that sense of peace through staring into a candle flame, or simply lying back on your bed and marvelling at the way in which you don't have to do anything to be alive in a given moment – it's as though you are being breathed.

<u>*Bandha* – Chapter 11</u>

Bandhas – energy locks – can be used in their more obvious, physical form as a way of finding certain qualities within your *asana* practice such as stability and lightness. Used judiciously they can lightly tone the inner musculature of your body such as your pelvic floor and core which support your internal organs and spine. As your practice progresses and your awareness becomes more finey attuned to energy, they can be used to retain and direct *prana* to a desired area.

<u>*Drishti* – Chapter 11</u>

Focusing your eyes and attention on a *drishti* – gaze point – is vital if you want to be able to balance in your *asana* practice when, for example, you are standing on one leg. So why use a *drishti* at other times during practice, when balance is relatively simple? Well, *drishti* is a great example of the crossover point between *dharana* (concentration) and *pratyahara* (withdrawal from the senses). When you totally focus one of your senses on a particular point, as we do with sight when we use a *drishti*, you withdraw it from other distractions. This, in turn, limits the distractions that your senses feed to your mind, and so your attention naturally draws in, to a more focused state of awareness. That in turn quietens your mind, and as we have learnt, '*yogah citta vrtti nirodhah*' – yoga is the cessation of the fluctuations of the mind.

Drishti is not only useful during mat-time; yoga practice is at its very best when we weave it into everyday life, and this mind-focusing tool is a valuable way of steadying mental activities and calming ourselves in times of stress. Taking a break from your computer screen to gaze at a stationary point outside the window or on a far wall both rests your eyes and helps you to gather your attention. Combine it with a few slow, full breaths and you elicit the relaxation response of your nervous system (chapter 6). This simple combination also makes for a lovely mini-meditation throughout your day when you're waiting for a bus, queueing in a shop, sitting in a café and so on. Far more beneficial than reflexively reaching for your phone!

What the Sutras Say

The consciousness becomes favourably
disposed, serene and benevolent by...

1.35 *Visayavati va pravrttih utpanna
manasah sthiti nibandhani*

...contemplating an object that helps to maintain
steadiness of mind and consciousness.

1.39 *Yathabhimata dhyanat va*

Or by meditating on any object conducive
to steadiness of consciousness.

Mudra – Chapter 11

Mudras – gestures – when used in formal practice help to direct your attention and *prana*, and thereby bring about certain psycho- energetic effects. Notice how each *mudra* makes you feel, and then enquire into yourself as to how you might use it to benefit everyday life. For example, if you find *yoni mudra* relaxing, you could place your hands on your lower abdomen to help you drift off to sleep. If you find that *jnana mudra* helps you to focus, you could use it any time your mind feels scattered. Remember, all of these practices are tools; once learnt, you have an incredible tool-kit of life-enhancing techniques with you at all times!

Yoga Nidra – Chapter 11

Yoga Nidra – yogic sleep - is an incredibly powerful practice for activating the myriad benefits of true, deep restorative relaxation, as well as accessing our own wisdom and insight, and even bringing about transformation in our lives (should that be desired). Delightfully, it's also an absolutely delicious way to spend a little time! The greatest obstacle to *yoga nidra*, in my experience, is a modern western fetishisation of busyness, and a societal sense that we should always be 'doing something' - it can feel extravagantly indulgent to give ourselves permission to simply lie down in the middle of the day and (to the onlooker at least) do nothing. However, I strongly encourage you to rebel against this notion and make time to lie back and follow a *yoga nidra* recording at least a couple of times a week! There are many available online – you'll find some on my website rocknrollyogi.com, and there are many wonderful ones on my *yoga nidra* teacher Uma Dinsmore-Tuli's site, yoganidranetwork.org.

Sankalpa – Chapter 11

Working with a *sankalpa* – highest vow - is an incredible effective way to make beneficial changes in our lives, from creating small shifts in behaviour to aligning with our *dharma* (true purpose). When your statement has been settled upon you can use in conjunction with *yoga nidra* to plant the seed in your subconscious mind; you can repeat it aloud or silently like a *mantra*; or you can simply maintain an awareness of it as you go about your daily business. Using a *sankalpa* in these multiple ways gives it many opportunites to really take root and move you in the direction of its calling.

Chanting, *Mantra* and *Kirtan* – Chapter 11

Although *kirtan* is a form of chanting which is most likely to take place in a group, there are many recordings available online if there is no group near you. You can choose to join in and sing along, or you might like to just listen with it in the background as you move through your day. Chanting and *mantra* can be solo practices, and you can use them both formally during your practice time, or throughout your day. Personally, chanting the *Gayatri mantra* in my car has carried me in good spirits through many a traffic jam which might otherwise have seen me getting stressed and irritable! And of course you don't have to do it out loud – simply mentally repeating the Universal *mantra* '*Om*' on each exhale is a fabulous way of connecting with something much larger than ourselves and bringing about a sense of peace.

<u>What the Sutras Say</u>

1.28 *Tajjapah tadarthabhavanam*

Om should be repeated constantly, with
feeling, realising its full significance.

1.29 *Tatah pratyakcetana adhigmah
api antaraya abhavanah ca*

Meditation on Om removes obstacles
to the mastery of the inner self.

Satsang – Chapter 11

Gathering in *satsang* – spiritual community – is a great way to meet yogi friends and explore the kinds of questions which there's not usually time for in a studio class. If no such group exists near you, you might suggest to your teacher that they consider starting one, or you can find several online around the world in a time zone which suits you.

Kriyas – Chapter 11

As part of a general yogic lifestyle, you might choose to adopt some of the *kriyas* – cleansing actions – into your routine. I find that *agni sara* and *nauli* - completely hollowing out the stomach and then churning it around - performed first thing in the morning on an empty stomach and followed by drinking a big glass of water, are extremely beneficial in maintaining healthy elimination. *Kapalbhati* – skull-shining breath - helps to clear my mind if I have brain fog or feel mentally overwhelmed; *neti* – nasal wash - is useful when I have hayfever; and *trataka* - candle gazing - is wonderful at bed time for combating jet-lag as it stimulates the pineal gland to produce the sleep-inducing hormone melatonin. *Basti* – enema or colonic irrigation - can be beneficial if you are doing a detox or experiencing disrupted bowel movements, but it's advisable to consult your doctor to rule out any medical issues if this is the case.

<u>*Chakras* – Chapter 12</u>

Understanding that the *chakras* – energy vortexes - describe how we use our *prana* – energy - in the world goes a long way to informing how we use knowledge of individual *chakras*. Chapter 12 gives you a number of suggestions for practices to work with a particular *chakra* depending on whether it is deficient or in excess. Remember also that the associated colours, musical tones, *mantras*, *mudras* and affirmations can be brought into your everyday life.

In addition, if a *chakra* is in excess it can often be beneficial to work with bringing energy to the *chakras* either side of it. For example, if you recognise in yourself a particularly domineering and aggressive attitude indicative of an excess of energy in *manipura* (solar plexus) *chakra*, it can be helpful to work with bringing more energy to the *svadhistana* (sacral) and *anahata* (heart) *chakras* using the practices suggested for their respective deficiencies.

<u>*Nadis* – Chapter 12</u>

Like the meridians in Chinese medicine, our *nadis* – energy channels - carry *prana* throughout the subtle energy body. The main ones with which we concern ourselves in practice are *sushumna*, *ida* and *pingala* – the central spinal channel, and the two which intertwine either side of it. *Ida* is related to the cooling lunar energy and we can physically work with it at the left nostril; *pingala* relates to the fiery solar energy and the right nostril. These two *nadis* switch in dominance throughout the day, usually every forty minutes or so. Alternate nostril breathing quickly reveals which one is currently dominant as that side will feel clearer. If you feel stressed or overly 'revved up', closing your right nostril and breathing through the left can help to rebalance you. Likewise, if you feel tired and lethargic and could use an energy boost, right-nostril breathing can pep you up.

<u>*Prana vayus* – Chapter 12</u>

Facilitating free-flowing *prana* in our bodies is one aim of a physical yoga practice. The *prana vayus* are the five major movements of energy within us, and in chapter 12 we touched on some of the practices which stimulate them.

You might like to focus your attention on detecting the direction of energy when you do one of these practices, and see if you can sense these movements of energy in yourself generally.

To recap:

Apana vayu describes a downward and outward motion of energy related to the lower body.

Prana vayu is an inward and upward movement describing the intake of energy, and is related to the body above the diaphragm, ie chest, shoulders, upper back, arms.

Samana vayu describes a horizontal and centripetal movement of energy, relating to the area between the navel and diaphragm.

Udana vayu is an upwards and outwards 'anti-gravity' motion, relating to the upper chest, throat, and head.

Vyana vayu is the outwardly circulating energy which moves energy from the centre to the periphery and helps the other *vayus* to move around the whole body.

Which of the vayus do you think is most stimulated by:

Bouncing on a trampoline?
Hula-hooping?
Squatting?
Dry skin brushing?
Taking big inhales?

This is useful information to bring to your general practice and life; however, as with the *chakras*, determining a *prana vayu* imbalance is best done in person by a qualified yoga therapist. They will observe your breath, movements, posture and demeanour to inform them as to the most beneficial practice for you as an individual.

Kleshas, Samskaras, and *Vikalpas* – Chapters 14 and 15

Yoga is a practice aimed at alleviating suffering. Although life presents us all with painful circumstances at times, much of our suffering originates either from our own mental state, or arises as a mental reaction to painful situations.

This is an important point on which Buddhism agrees with yoga philosophy – our futile tendency to want things to be a certain way, to cling on to some experiences and reject others, and resist life as it is, creates suffering (which is optional) on top of pain (which may be unavoidable). Pain is the first arrow which may come from elsewhere; but our lack of skill in handling it means that we often shoot the second arrow at ourselves.

We are only human, and our psychological make-up dictates that we are subject to our *kleshas* – the mental afflictions of misunderstanding, mistaken identity, attachments, aversions, and fear. From the day we are born we accumulate *samskaras* – impressions – about the world, and we make up stories and mental constructs – *vikalpas* – about how life works and how things 'ought' to be.

Developing awareness of our own psychological habits and tendencies is vital if we are to loosen these mental afflictions which keep us in the bondage of self-created suffering. All of yoga's practices lead us to a greater steadiness of mind and the ability to see a little more clearly – it's like wiping dirt from our lenses so that we can see what's actually happening rather than just staring at the dirt and perceiving that to be the whole picture. Combine the practice with a keen awareness of your personal *kleshas*, *samskaras*, and *vikalpas*, and you will find yourself firmly on the path to a far greater sense of peace and freedom within yourself. It's not so much that a steady mind and keen awareness will eradicate these tendencies – again, we are only human – but that deepening our self-knowledge and expanding our awareness gradually loosens the constraints that keep us jailed within our own minds.

<u>*Dharma* and the *Purusharthas* – Chapter 16</u>

Dharma is the organising principle of the Universe, and our individual *dharma* is where we fit into that. By fulfilling our Earthly duties to ourselves, the people around us, and the wider world, we live our true purpose.

This is one of the four driving principles of human life known as the *purusharthas*. The others are:

Artha - the drive to meet our practical needs and responsibilities.

Kama - the drive for pleasure.

Moksha - the drive for spiritual liberation.

Different *purusharthas* predominate at different stages of life – for example, someone in their forties who is raising a family will probably spend a lot of time working on *artha*; someone who is older and no longer bound by the demands of young children may find themselves drawn to the spiritual exploration and contemplation of *moksha*. However, all of these desires are with us throughout our lifespans, and it makes for a happier and more balanced life if we can honour each of them in some way each day. This is a perfect opportunity for a little *svadhyaya* (self-enquiry):

- How am I honouring *dharma* in my life?

- How am I honouring *artha* in my life?
- How am I honouring *kama* in my life?
- How am I honouring *moksha* in my life?

There are many different paths and subdivisions of yoga - these are the main types which you might meet.

Raja yoga is the 'royal yoga' of Patanjali's Yoga Sutras, and encompasses several of the other schools. Although *asana* (postures) are mentioned briefly, the emphasis is on meditation and the chief actions (*kriyas)* are *tapas* (self-discipline/zealousness in practice), *svadhyaya* (self-enquiry and study), and *Ishvara-pranidhana* (surrender to the Divine).

Jnana yoga is the yoga of wisdom or knowledge, whose primary practices are meditation, study and self-enquiry.

Tantra yoga is sorely misunderstood in the west as a sexual sect, largely thanks to new-age distortions of a tiny part of Tantrik practice which is limited to extremely advanced practitioners. The overwhelming majority of what gets called Tantra these days is actually new-age spiritualised sexuality. (There's nothing wrong with that in itself, but we should be aware of the distinction – there are some questionable individuals around who take advantage of the misunderstanding – indeed, they may well be subject to the misunderstanding themselves – with damaging consequences.) There are very few surviving teachers of classical Tantra, which is to do with energy and Consciousness. The word Tantra means 'the wisdom that saves', and it is a profoundly life-affirming world view which teaches from the premise that we can find liberation IN the world, not FROM the world. There is a strong emphasis on deities as representations of different aspects of the one Divine nature (which is comprised of energy - *Shakti* - and Consciousness - *Shiva*). The chief practices of its yoga are *mantra* (word or phrase), *yantra* (divine geometry), meditation, visualisation, *kriya* (purification rituals), *asana* (postures) and *pranayama* (breathwork).

Tantra is a vast and fascinating subject. If it interests you, some respected teachers whose work you may like to investigate include Pandit Rajmani Tigunait, Rod Stryker, Sally Kempton, and Christopher D. Wallis.

'Tantra Illuminated' by Christopher D. Wallis is an excellent book which explains and demystifies the subject very well.

Karma yoga is about doing the right thing, non-violence, and mindfulness, as well as selfless service – helpful actions with no attachment to or expectation of results or reward.

Bhakti yoga is the yoga of devotion, and includes offerings and ritual, *mantra*, and meditation on one of many deities.

Kundalini yoga is a topic which has a lot of confusion around it, and there are many different definitions. *Kundalini* itself is a form of energy, which is variously described by different philosophies as abiding as a coiled snake at the base of the spine waiting to be awakened; or as a higher and lower *kundalini* at the crown of the head and base of the spine which must meet to reach integration; or as a blockage to the flow of *prana* along the *sushumna nadi* which must be burned up. The concept of *kundalini* is first discovered in Tantrik texts, and Tantrik yoga works a lot with this energy.

The *Kundalini* yoga which you may see classes for, often identifiable by teachers wearing white clothing and a turban, was formulated in the 20th century by a teacher called Yogi Bhajan. It includes vigorous rhythmic movements, *pranayama*, and chanting.

Hatha yoga is to do with the physical body and counts *asana*, *pranayama*, meditation, *bandha* (energy seals), *mudra* (gestures, usually with the hands), and *kriya* amongst its practices. Its central text is the Hatha Yoga Pradipika, written around the 13th century.The aim of *Hatha* yoga is to release, strengthen and balance the structure of the body, to enable prana to flow and circulate freely. The vast majority of western yoga falls under the umbrella of

Hatha yoga, and it encompasses the familiar styles such as Iyengar, *Ashtanga, Vinyasa* and so on.

Several of the familiar styles today descend from a teacher called Sri T Krishnamacharya (1888-1989), who is often referred to as the father of modern yoga. He had a number of noted students who went on to popularise yoga in the west, including his son TKV Desikachar, BKS Iyengar, Sri K Pattabhi Jois, Indra Devi and AG Mohan.

What to expect in your class

This is a brief overview of what you might expect from some popular types of class: however, every teacher has their own unique style, so explore. If you don't connect with something the first time, be open to trying the same style of class with a different teacher.

Hatha

Although *Hatha* describes many forms of physical yoga, it is common to see '*Hatha*' offered as a style of class – this typically denotes a style of teaching which emphasises *asana* and *pranayama*, usually without the flowing '*vinyasa*' linking postures. Classes can vary from physically very gentle to quite demanding.

Vinyasa

A *vinyasa* class is characterised by a flowing style, with a '*vinyasa*' movement comprising *Chaturanga Dandasana* (Low Plank), *Urdhva Mukha Svanasana* (Upward Facing Dog) and *Adho Mukha Svanasana* (Downward Facing Dog) forming the transition between postures.

Iyengar

Iyengar classes focus heavily on detailed alignment, tend to use several props, and often have the student hold postures for longer than in other styles.

Ashtanga

Ashtanga is a physically challenging, dynamic practice which follows a set sequence of postures. There are six series of sequences, although few practitioners progress beyond the primary and second series. Some classes are 'led', meaning that the teacher verbally guides you through the whole practice; others are 'Mysore' style, when practioners work through the sequence at their own pace and receive individual support from the teacher as he or she moves around the room (which is like a private class within the energy of a group). The emphasis is on *asana* with *Ujjayi pranayama*, *bandhas*, and *drishti*. There are traditionally a lot of physical adjustments and hands-on assists from the teacher in this style, and of course you always have the right to request only verbal suggestions if you want to practise without being touched.

Ashtanga means eight limbs – just like the eight limbs which we met in chapter 2. Most classes that you see advertised as Ashtanga will refer to the vigorous style popularised by Pattabhi Jois, but it's worth clarifying with the teacher whether they mean this, or a more traditional philosophy based class.

Yin

In a Yin class each pose is held for a long time, going progressively deeper into a stretch as the body releases tension from muscles and fascia. Much of the class will generally be seated or lying down, as the 'yin' aspect describes a passive approach to this release, but the class can still be challenging, as we learn to stay in uncomfortable (though they should never be painful) places.

Restorative

In a Restorative class, the body is fully supported by props such as bolsters and blankets. In common with Yin, each pose is held for several minutes; however, unlike Yin the objective is not a deep stretch, and any such sensation should be mild and diminish over time. The purpose is to allow the very deepest layers of the body's musculature, such as the postural muscles of the core and spine, to release tension and to bring about a feeling of deep inner relaxation and peace in the body, energy and mind.

Pre-Natal

As the name suggests, pre-natal yoga is for expectant mothers to prepare for birth and establish a bond with their baby.

Bikram and hot yoga

Hot yoga is typically practised in a room heated to between 34 and 42 degrees Celcius. Many practitioners enjoy the idea that they are detoxing through sweating heavily, and the increased flexibility of the body that the heat provides. Bikram is such a form with a set sequence which was designed by Bikram Choudhury in the 1970s.

<u>Beer yoga, goat yoga and beyond… is it really yoga?</u>

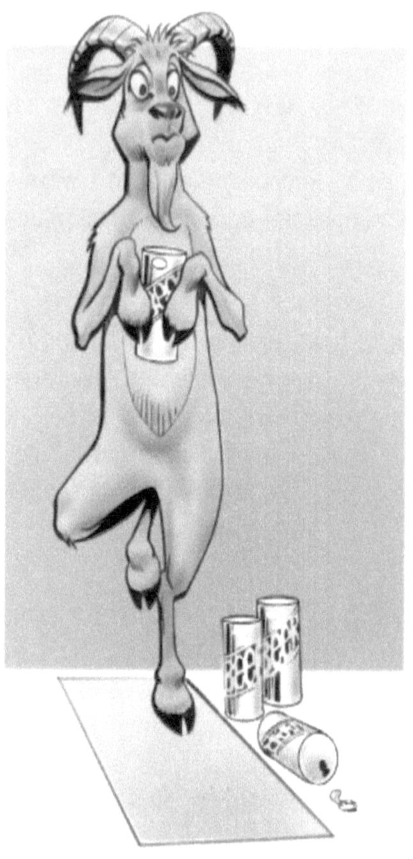

A lot of contemporary forms calling themselves yoga have sprung up in recent years, and whilst they might be a fun way to spend some time, they're not traditional. There's an argument in favour of them from the point of view of 'whatever gets you through the door'; we all come to yoga in our own time and our own way, and if someone enjoys their special edition class enough to get curious about more authentic yoga then it might serve as an entry point. If someone needs some fun and connection in their life and they enjoy their time at that class and make new friends, then really, what's wrong with that? The discovery of joy and connection is, after all, a large part of practice – and yoga is not only what we do on the mat, but how we live our lives.

That said, it's important to understand that yoga is a profound practice to alleviate suffering by freeing us from the vagaries of our minds and find Self-realisation; and so calling these classes yoga is a distortion of ancient wisdom. Beer, goats, and so on might be fun, but perhaps we need a new name for them instead of yoga!

<u>Yoga Therapy</u>

Yoga Therapy is an active, complementary, holistic therapy which empowers the individual to participate in their own healing.

It's 'active' because, rather than being done *to* you (like massage for example), the client takes an active role and does the practice themselves, at first in session under the guidance of the therapist, and then at home by themselves on an agreed regular basis. This might be as little as three minutes a day, but simplicity and regularity are key when it comes to a therapeutic yoga practice.

'Complementary' (as opposed to alternative), means that yoga therapy is an adjunct to, not an alternative for, conventional medicine. A yoga therapist should never contradict medical opinion and treatment or advise a client to come off medication, and the therapist uses a medical diagnosis (if there is one) as an initial means of understanding what the client might be experiencing and a signpost to know what *not* to do (ie what practices are contraindicated) so that they can keep the client safe. Yoga therapy is a wonderful support to whatever treatment the client may be undergoing, and although we never interfere with medical prescriptions, the client often finds that in time their symptoms are alleviated significantly enough that their doctor can reassess their dosage.

Finally, 'holistic' means that there is no 'in case of x, do y' in yoga therapy - the client is treated as a *whole*, rather than as their complaint. Remember the *koshas* that we explored in chapter 1? A yoga therapist seeks to bring all aspects of a client's being into a more balanced state, so improving their whole personal state and creating a favourable environment in which to thrive.

*A*yurveda is an ancient Indian system for attaining optimal health which complements yoga beautifully. The basis of *Ayurvedic* theory is that we are each made up of the five elements - earth, water, fire, air and space – in different combinations. The combinations of these elements are called the *doshas*, and they are:

Pitta: fire and water
Kapha: earth and water
Vata: air and space

Pitta creates light and heat, as well as the energies of digestion (on physical, mental and spiritual levels) and transformation. It manifests as qualities of motivation, courage, and vitality. Physically it relates to the stomach and small intestine, and the eyes. If it's out of balance it can lead to an excess of psychological drive and overwork, digestive disorders and inflammation.

Kapha creates steadiness and hydration, and the energies of stability and devotion. It manifests as qualities of love, caring and dependability. Physically it relates to the chest and bodily fluids such as plasma and mucus, and the nose and tongue. If it's out of balance it can lead to laziness, attachment, and lack of motivation.

Vata creates movement and speed, and the energies of mobility and adaptability. It manifests as creativity, enthusiasm and responsiveness. Physically it relates to the large intestine, skin and ears, and air in spaces such as joints and bones. If it's out of balance it can lead to excess gas within the body, exhaustion, and nervous disorders.

Although we all have at least a little of each element, we can each be described as having a predominance of one of these *doshas* according to our individual physical and psychological make-up. Many people have a combination of two predominant *doshas*, and a few people have the three in equal measure and are descibed as tri-*doshic*. No type is superior or inferior – they all have their benefits and their drawbacks.

Our individual *dosha* constituency is determined at the start of life and stays with us throughout. This is called our *prakriti*.

It's common for us to be out of balance and for one of the *doshas* to be in excess. This, our imbalance, is called our *vikruti*.

<u>Classic *dosha* types</u>

A typical *pitta* predominant person tends to be of medium size, with strong muscles which build up easily. Their skin is often warm and possibly ruddy, their eyes bright and light, their hair fine and soft. Their movements are focused and deliberate. They are very driven, tenacious 'go go go' types, keen to take on more and be challenged (and can tend towards burnout as a result) and they generally sleep well. If you want something done effectively and efficiently, get a *pitta* person involved!

A typically *kapha* predominant person is of a larger, heavier build; tall, with smooth and flexible joint movements. They tend to have thick, lustrous hair and large eyes and are often quite beautiful. They are fond of relaxation and sleep heavily. Their demeanour is slow and steady, relaxed and easy-going. As a welcoming, chilled out companion, a *kapha* type is hard to beat!

A typical *vata* predominant person might be either quite small or tall, of fine build, with hair that is brittle and skin that is dry. They often feel cold as their circulation can be weak, and their joints often crack. Their movements are restless, their sleep is light and their energy can be erratic and scattered. *Vata* types are often highly creative and intuitive – many artistic people have a lot of *vata*.

If someone is a combination of two *doshas*, that is expressed by placing the slightly more dominant one first – for example, I am *pitta-vata*, my friend is *vata-pitta* - and it's possible to tend more towards one *dosha* physically and another psychologically.

Knowing our own *dosha prakriti* – which is fixed – means that we can support ourselves in the best possible way through a tailored diet and lifestyle. To give an example, one premise of an *Ayurvedic* diet is that 'more begets more', so a highly fiery *pitta* person who eats a lot of hot and spicy food will exacerbate their *pitta* and create imbalance. They would be better advised to eat cooling salads and raw foods. A *kapha* type will be aggravated by heavy, oily foods and will create more balance with light dishes such as steamed vegetables. A *vata* will increase *vata* with food straight from the refrigerator or dry, airy things like rice cakes, and will be balanced by warming, grounding foods like soup or casseroles.

A quiz such as the one on the next page can give you a strong idea of what your own constitution might be. Sometimes it's immediately obvious, if you have a very predominant *dosha*; with other people determining their *prakriti* can be an intricate process and even an *Ayurvedic* doctor may want to see a patient a few times before they are sure. They can also determine where we are out of balance – our *vikruti* – and this is what is commonly addressed by *Ayurvedic* treament, which encompasses herbs, diet, lifestyle management, and can usefully inform the type of yoga practice which is most suitable for you at different times of your life. *Ayurveda* can help us to reduce *doshic* excesses, and to live in a way which best supports our individual constitution.

Determine Your *Dosha*

Grade your responses as:
0 - doesn't describe me at all
1 - describes me a little
2 - describes me fairly well
3 - describes me very well

	Vata	*Pitta*	*Kapha*
Physical build	thin, slight	medium, well-muscled	large, heavy
Height	tall or short	average	medium or tall
Skin	dry, thin, flaky	warm, ruddy	smooth, oily
Joints	cracking, stiff	average, loose	flexible, large
Eyes	small, darting, hazel	medium, piercing, light	large, white, lustrous
Hair	dry, thin, wavy, coarse	fine, soft, straight	thick, oily, abundant

Nails	thin, brittle	medium, pink	large, thick, pale, soft
Circulation	poor, variable	good	moderate
Appetite	erratic	high	moderate but constant
Movement	restless, fidgety	moderate, purposeful	slow, steady
Temperament	vivacious, erratic	driven, tenacious	easy-going, content
Activities	creative, intuitive	technical, political	business, social, family
Energy	erratic, hyperactive	moderate-high, driven	steady, good stamina
Sleep	light, restless	moderate, falls asleep easily	heavy, slow to wake
Total			

Ayurveda is a big topic and an in-depth explanation is beyond the scope of this book. For further reading I suggest Textbook of *Ayurveda* : Volume 1 - Fundamental Principles of *Ayurveda* by Vasant Lad.

Chapter 20 – Other words you might hear and what they mean

Yogi/yogini - A *yogi*, strictly speaking, is someone who has reached Self-realisation through yoga; but in modern day use a *yogi* or *yogini* is simply someone who practises yoga. *Yogi* is the masculine form, *yogini* the feminine, although it's common to use *yogi* for all genders (much like actor and actress).

Shala - House or home, used in reference to a place where we practise yoga – a 'house of yoga'.

Sadhana - Our *sadhana* is our practice.

Sadhaka - A *sadhaka* is one who practises.

Shraddha – Deep and abiding faith; 'that which is placed in the heart.'

Namaste - A greeting most often heard at the end of a yoga class, *namaste* means 'the light within me recognises and honours the light within you'. It can be said as a hello or a farewell.

Om - pronounced A-U-M – the primordial sound, the sound of Universal Consciousness, life, the unmanifest cosmos. The Yoga Sutra describes it as the sound on which by meditating we can realise *samadhi*.

Om Shanti Shanti Shanti - This means '*Om*, peace peace peace'. We meet this phrase at the end of each of the Upanishads, and you'll often hear it chanted in class. It's an intention, wish, or blessing for peace within ourselves, peace to those whom we know, and peace to the wider world and Universe.

Hari Om Tat Sat - *Hari* means 'the manifest universe', ie all matter. *Om* represents the unmanifest Universal Consciousness. *Tat* means that, and *Sat* means ultimate truth. So '*Hari Om Tat Sat*' means 'the manifest, the Consciousness, that is truth'. This greeting reminds us of who we really are; that our bodies are made of stardust, our Selves are sparks of pure Consciousness. This is the essence of yoga.

Sat Nam - This is a universal mantra which is sometimes used as a way to focus the mind in order to enter into a state of meditation. It means 'true name' – inviting us back to the truth of who we really are – not Sally or John, but the formless Consciousness beyond all mind and labels.

Guru - This is a word which carries with it some difficulties, due to the abuse of power by some *gurus*. It can mean simply, 'teacher'. It can mean 'one who leads from darkness to light'. It can refer to the *guru*-principle – the power of awakend awareness. And it can refer, sometimes problematically, to the idea of the *guru* on a pedestal, who is infallible and should not be challenged or questioned.

Shiva/Shakti - *Shiva* and *Shakti* are (very simplistically) the masculine and feminine principles at play in the Universe, and are more commonly found in *Tantrik* teachings. *Shiva* represents pure Consciousness, *Shakti* represents energy.

Mandala - A geometric, usually round, arrangement of symbols which is often used to focus concentration and establish a sacred space.

Yantra - A graphic geometric depiction of energy from the *Tantrik* tradition, usually square. They are associated with the energy and qualities of a particular deity – they are the visual representation of that deity, just as a *mantra* is the sound form - and *trataka* gazing and meditation upon them is used to manifest their powers.

As we come towards the end of this book's journey together, I hope that you have discovered a sense of how practical this ancient wisdom of yoga really is, and how it is just as applicable to modern life as it was when it was first committed to text. Personally, yoga has enriched, informed, and improved every aspect of my life since I first stumbled upon it. I have yet to meet the situation which it cannot illuminate and guide! Yoga is a vast treasure trove of universally applicable life wisdom, which brings greater freedom and peace to every aspect of our experience.

The *asanas* are a wonderful, intrinsically valuable part of yoga; nonetheless, their physical appeal has sometimes led to them being somewhat over-represented in the general western understanding of what yoga is. Yoga is a comprehensive methodology for living well and looking after all aspects of ourselves. It is the cessation of fluctuations of our minds, to thereby alleviate our suffering and discover a state of Self-realisation. Our yoga mats are the laboratory - it's when we step off them and into the world that we truly have the opportunity to live our yoga in everyday life, in our actions, encounters, and relationships.

It is my heartfelt wish that this book helps you to enrich your own life and find that state of freedom – of yoga - which is ever present within you.

The light in me recognises and honours the light in you.

Namaste.

Glossary of terms used in this book

Abhinivesa – insecurity; fear (esp. of death - one of the five kleshas)
Ahimsa – non-violence (one of the five yamas)
Ahamkara – ego
Ajna – third eye chakra
Alabdhabhumikatva – lack of perseverance (one of the nine obstacles)
Alasya – laziness (one of the nine obstacles)
Anahata – heart chakra (lit: unstruck)
Ananda – bliss
Anandamaya – bliss sheath (of koshas)
Anavasithatvani - regression (one of the nine obstacles)
Anjali (mudra) – prayer hands
Annamaya – food sheath (of koshas)
Apana – downward movement of energy within the subtle body (one of the five prana yayus); bodily waste
Aparigraha – non-grasping; letting go (one of the five yamas)
Asana – posture; seat (one of the eight limbs)
Ashtanga – eight limbs
Asmita – misidentification (esp. with ego - one of the five kleshas)
Asteya – non-stealing (one of the five yamas)
Avidya – misapprehension; spiritual ignorance (one of the five kleshas)
Avirati – overindulgence (one of the nine obstacles)
Ayurveda – holistic lifestyle science
Bandha – lock, seal (esp. energy)
Basti – enema
Bhakti - devotion
Bija - seed
Brahmacharya – continence (esp. sexual - one of the five yamas)
Brahmari (pranayama) – humming bee breath
Brantidarshana – wrong view; illusion (one of the nine obstacles)
Buddhi - intelligence
Chakra – wheel (ie of energy)
Dharana – concentration (one of the eight limbs)
Dharma – life's purpose
Dhauti - cleansing

Dhyana – meditation (one of the eight limbs)
Dosha – constitutional type
Drishti – gaze point
Ekagrata – single-pointed
Guna – quality of nature
Guru – teacher
Hasta – hand
Hatha – yoga comprising physical practices
Ida – lunar energy channel
Ishvara-pranidhana – surrender to the Divine (one of the five niyamas)
Jalandhara (bandha) – throat lock
Japa - repetition
Jnana – wisdom; knowledge beyond book learning
Jnanendriya - sense organ
Kama - pleasure
Karma – action; Universal law of cause and effect
Karmendriya – organ of action
Kirtan – group chanting, usually with music
Klesha – affliction; cause of suffering
Kosha – sheath; body
Kriya – action
Kshipta – scattered (ie mind)
Kundalini – coiled energy which travels along central energy channel upon awakening
Manas – mind
Mandala – geometric shape for concentration, usually circular
Manipura – solar plexus chakra
Manomaya – mind sheath (one of the five koshas)
Mantra – sacred phrase
Mudra – gesture, usually of hands
Mudha – dull; unclear (ie state of mind)
Mula – root
Muladhara – root chakra
Nadi – energy channel
Nadi shodhana – type of pranayama, alternate nostril breathing
Nauli – abdominal churning
Neti – nasal cleansing

Nidra - sleep
Nirodha – suspension; stillness
Niyama – personal observance
Om – primordial sound; sacred sound of the Universe
Pada – chapter (of Sutras); foot
Patanjali – great sage, author of Yoga Sutras
Pingala – solar energy channel
Pramada – negligence; carelessness (one of the nine obstacles)
Prana – life-force; energy; (also one of the five prana yayus)
Pranamaya – energy body (one the five koshas)
Prakriti - matter
Pratyahara – withdrawal of / from the senses (one of the eight limbs)
Purusha – pure Consciousness
Raga – attachment (one of the five kleshas)
Rajas – quality of vibrancy, motion, dynamism (one of the three gunas)
Sadhaka - practitioner
Sadhana – practice
Sahasrara – crown chakra
Sama – same; equal
Samadhi – merging into unity with the Universe (one of the eight limbs)
Samana – centripetal movement of energy within the body (one of the five prana yayus)
Samsaya – doubt (one of the nine obstacles)
Sankalpa – highest vow; intention
Sanskrit – language of yoga
Santosha – contentment (one of the five niyamas)
Satsang – gathering of like-minded people; sitting with yogic community for discussion
Sattva – quality of clarity, luminosity, illumination (one of the three gunas)
Satya – truthfulness (one of the five yamas)
Shakti – feminine energy of the Universe
Shala – space where one practices
Shanti - peace
Sharira – body
Shiva – masculine energy of the Universe
Sitali – type of pranayama with rolled tongue
Sthira - steady

Styana – inertia (one of the nine obstacles)
Sukha – comfortable; sweet
Sushumna – central energy channel of the subtle body corresponding with spinal cord
Sutra – thread
Svadhistana – sacral chakra
Svadhyaya – self-study; self-enquiry (one of the five niyamas)
Tamas – quality of dullness, heaviness, inertia
Tantra – system of philosophy related to yoga
Tapas – burning zeal; disipline
Tattva – principle of nature
Trataka – gazing at an object
Udana – upward movement of energy within the body (one of the five prana yayus)
Uddiyana – stomach bandha (energy lock) – 'upward flying'
Ujjayi – type of pranayama with constricted glottis
Vayu – movement of energy within the subtle body ('wind')
Vikalpa – mental construct
Viloma – type of pranayama (ladder breath)
Vinyasa – movement; flowing style of yoga
Vishuddhi – throat chakra
Vrtti – fluctuation (ie of mind)
Vyadhi – sickness (one of the nine obstacles)
Vyana – circulatory movement of energy within the subtle body (one of the five prana yayus)
Yama – universal observance
Yantra – geometric depiction of energy
Yoni – female reproductive organs

Yogic texts which you might like to explore

The Yoga Sutras – I like BKS Iyengar's translation for its clarity, and Bernard Bouanchaud's for its poetic self-enquiry explorations for using the Sutras in our own lives.
The Bhagavad Gita – I like Eknath Easwaran's translation.
The Upanishads – Again, I like Eknath Easwaran's translation.
Hatha Yoga Pradipika
Gheranda Samhita